ON THE WINGS OF SUCCESS

ISBN: 978-1720790600

DEDICATION

This book is gratefully dedicated to my husband and my family, who encouraged me to continue to pursue my vision of writing this book. Thank you for believing in me! This is also for anyone who has been affected by Fetal Alcohol Spectrum Disorder, and for those who work tirelessly to continue to learn and educate about FASD. A very special thank you goes out to all who participated by volunteering to share their stories. You are all so special and experts on this topic!

TABLE OF CONTENTS

WHAT IS FETAL ALCOHOL SPECTRUM DISORDER?

Fetal Alcohol Spectrum Disorder (FASD) is the result of prenatal exposure to alcohol. During pregnancy, whatever the mother consumes, so does her baby! There is no known safe amount of alcohol a mother can drink during her pregnancy, so it is well advised that she abstain from drinking any alcohol to avoid causing harm to the unborn baby. ***Fetal Alcohol Spectrum Disorder is 100% preventable!*** It is a life long disability and the effects are irreversible.

Below are a few signs and symptoms of FASD. The Fetal Alcohol Spectrum Disorder umbrella has different terms of FASD and ARND to

4

describe the varying symptoms. ***To determine a thorough diagnosis, please consult a physician.***

Fetal Alcohol Spectrum Disorder (FASD):

FASD comprises a multi-layered array of neurodevelopmental and physical disabilities as which are the result of pre-natal exposure to alcohol. Neurodevelopmental deficiencies include abnormalities affecting the ability to self regulate behavior, thoughts, emotions and experiencing difficulties learning due to the pre-natal exposure to alcohol.

Identifying physical features can include:

- Smooth philtrum (the groove between the nose and upper lip)
- Thin upper lip
- Small eyes
- Upturned nose
- Small head size
- Low body weight

- Vision or hearing problems
- Deficiencies with the heart, kidneys, or bones
- Central nervous system deficiencies

Alcohol-Related Neurodevelopmental Disorder (ARND):

ARND falls under the umbrella of FASD which includes the same multi-layered range of disabilities seen in FASD. Abnormalities in neurodevelopment includes the inability to self regulate their emotions and behavior, due to the pre-natal exposure to alcohol.

Behavioral symptoms can include:

- Attention problems
- Learning problems
- Dysmaturity
- Difficulty in school
- Memory problems; forgetting how to do something they have done before

- Complications forming or maintaining relationships with peers
- Temper tantrums; mood swings
- Hyperactive, impulsive behavior
- Trusting too easily which can leave them vulnerable to dangerous situations
- Unable to understand consequences (cause and effect)
- Co-fabulation (lying)
- Drug and/or alcohol addictions

Interdependent resources and community services which provide positive routine, structure and support can be critical to assist those who are affected by FASD. Supports can enable their ability to live a fulfilling life while building self-esteem and a confident sense of self.

AUTHOR'S NOTE
INTRODUCTION

I am by no means, a writer! The idea of this book came from a research paper that I needed to write for a course I was taking at the time. We expect to be able to find whatever we need from the internet. I was shocked to discover much of the information I found online drew a very bleak future for anyone who had suffered the effects of alcohol in utero. On the third day of researching and growing increasingly frustrated with what I was finding, I had a thought pop into my head. "

I'm going to write a book of success stories about people who have FASD!"

This idea was the beginning of a very real, informative and humbling learning journey. I am honoured to be able to write this book about these wonderful people who have some incredible life stories to share. My hope, with having compiled these stories, is to highlight the positive in the world of FASD. I have learned and heard first hand how resilient, forgiving and persistent their spirit can be. They have shared their creativity, talents, shown their ability to laugh easily and their big hearts. Life can be tough for anyone who has FASD, but these difficulties are often faced with determination and optimism. With these stories of their personal successes, I aspire it to instill a better understanding of how society can learn to assist them better. FASD may be a disability, but it hasn't stopped them from achieving goals and being everything that most research says they will never be. I wrote this book to celebrate their accomplishments and personal triumphs.

Without further ado, I hope you enjoy reading their stories.

CHAPTER 1
Rebecca T.

I was adopted at birth from New Jersey. My parents adopted me through Bethany Christian Services, which is an adoption agency. My adoptive parents had a baby that they lost at five days old. She was a preemie, so after she was born it, they turned to adoption, and they got a phone call nine months, or maybe around a year after she passed away. They already had a son, who was four years old at the time. They got a call about me, and they drove to New Jersey. They held me, and they learned what they could about me. New Jersey has closed records. So, all they were given was the date of birth, the first name, and that there may have been drinking during the pregnancy, but that she wasn't an alcoholic. That is what they wrote on this paper that they gave my parents. They said I was

10

healthy. My parents made the decision, "Let's go adopt her." I went home with them at four weeks old, on Valentine's Day, actually. I went home, and I got really sick. I had constant ear infections, like every week. I had bronchitis. I didn't eat much for the first eighteen months. I was diagnosed with failure to thrive. The doctors didn't know why. That piece of paper said there may have been drinking, but she wasn't an alcoholic. Thinking back, I think they lied on the paperwork, to try to get me to home. My birth mom lied too. I have photos of me as an infant. They brought me to a pediatrician, and the pediatrician looked at me, and I had facial features of Fetal Alcohol Syndrome. I have a flat philtrum, and my nose was flatter. My eyes were....something with the eyes the doctor said was characteristic. My face was flatter than it should be. My eyes were a little droopy. That's what it was. He didn't diagnose me formally. He said it could be. Maybe not. Plus I had failure to thrive. So, it was in the back of their mind, but back in 1980, nobody ever even followed through meaning the doctor said the words, and then it was forgotten about. So, I was in the hospital, and they checked me for cystic fibrosis, cancer...everything, and everything came back negative. Around eighteen months, I started to eat. My ears started to get better, and I started to thrive.

My parents are incredible! I will say, as the studies have shown, that the environment that you are raised in if you have Fetal Alcohol Syndrome makes such a difference. I was successful. I did wonderful in school. The only thing I struggled with which got worse as I got older is writing, outlines, organization, remembering dates, and times. Math, I stink at. I can read really well. I struggled with things that a lot of people do! So, just thought it was me! I was successful, and I got straight A's, or 4.0's. I was very good in school. I got into college, and I wanted to be speech therapist. That's where it fell apart, because I did great in classroom, but then I had to go student teach. To be a teacher, or a speech therapist even, it's so abstract. You teach kids different, and I couldn't figure it out, how to apply different methods of learning to the kids I taught. It was too abstract for me. Writing reports....I thought they made sense, but they were all garbled, and not organized at all. In 2002, I got a Bachelors in Speech Therapy...barely! My school grades were wonderful, but I barely passed student teaching because it was too overwhelming for me. I went for my Masters. I thought ok! I struggled with student teaching. I struggled with writing. Who doesn't? Because again, my Fetal Alcohol is really mild. Extremely! I have been blessed as to how mild it is. The bachelors is an awesome accomplishment! I went for my Masters, and I failed! I student taught, and it's a lot harder at that level. They just said that your lesson plans aren't making sense. You're not helping the kids. And then I had a report writing class, and I couldn't cohesively write a report. So, they failed me, which was devastating. It was fine. I was able to work in preschool, with little kids as a speech therapist for five years. I just had to have somebody sign off on my work, and I didn't have to write big reports, at all. In the real world, you don't have to. You can just write little notes here and there. I made progress, and I didn't have anybody looking over my shoulder. Less anxiety! Overcoming the disappointment from failing the master's program was hard. Actually, it is still very bad. It's been over ten years, and I am bitter about it to this day. But I don't stay in one place. If something bad happens, I have the ability to move forward pretty quickly. I don't know why. It could be because my brain doesn't allow me to stop what I'm doing. I was hurt, and I was upset. But I knew I had to move forward because I was getting married, and I wanted a family and so I kind of just trudged forward. But the feelings are still there. They were dealt with kind of, but…..I moved forward, and I worked at a daycare for a little bit, and now, I work at State Farm Insurance. I'm a representative, and I've been there for ten years. I love it! I'm good at it! The only thing I'm not good at which they help me with is report writing. They know that I have a learning disability. They don't really know what it is, or they might. I don't know. But they help me. My boss helps me, and I'm ok with it. They are willing to help me to succeed. It is a lot of memorization, which I am good at. I don't forget phone numbers. I don't forget numbers. I am very good at that, and I am very good at….I can be very detailed when I write. Details are good for me. It's just going in outline form. It's that organizational piece. It's the same with my everyday life. If I don't write things down, I forget the simplest things. Like, when my child was an infant, I would leave the house without the diaper bag. But, everyone does! That's a new mom thing too! It's weird, because I feel odd saying I have Fetal Alcohol, because I am one of the very, very mild cases. A lot of my issues, a lot of people that don't have it struggle with. I am blessed.

What prompted me to get tested is my adoptive mom were close, but we clash, just like every mother and daughter. We had a huge fight. I don't even know what it was over. I was visiting her. I went home, and in the mail, she got this pamphlet from the adoption agency that they adopted me from. It was about Fetal Alcohol Spectrum Disorder. She was like, what is this? She started reading it. She called me on the phone crying. She was like you have so many of these symptoms, and I think this is why you have organizational issues, and I think this why you have this issue, and that issue. I go from zero to sixty very quickly. I have no patience. So, she says this, and everything made sense to me.

It was 2013, I found my birth Mom. She passed away. I found out who she was because I was on Classmates.com. I knew her date of birth, so I started doing research. I knew she lived in New Jersey. I found a photo. I knew her first name. I knew she had a polish last name. So, I found her, and she looked just like me. I was happy to find her, because I always wanted to know who she was. My parents stood behind me 100% until I found her. Before I knew she was dead, they told me they knew I had to find her, but they were scared because they didn't know what was coming next. They were terrified! They will never say that! They will say we weren't scared! We trusted you! We knew you had to do it! But, just the way they acted. I mean, I would be scared if I were them! So, I found out, and then I found people that knew her. She passed away.

Everyone that knew her said that she drank the entire time she was pregnant with me. She drank heavily. I have a brother too, that I have never met who is ten years older than me. She drank with him too. I think I found him. I didn't know I had a brother until somebody that knew her told me. He was put up for adoption. I think I found him, but he doesn't want anything to do with it. We have parted ways, because I have to respect that. So, yeah! She drank a lot. She died from her liver. She died at 58, and her liver was …..I got an autopsy report, and her liver was decayed, and she died with a blood alcohol level of 0.48 or something like that. She was an alcoholic. It was sad, and I am sad for her, because I never got to know her. But she was an orphan herself, I found out. Her brother, who I met, she was born, and placed in an orphanage, and lived in foster care until she was 18. She had nobody. She didn't know what to do, so she drank. It made sense.

So, now my Mom and I think I have Fetal Alcohol. Now, I take it upon myself to find a geneticist to test me at 34 years old. There is nobody in the area except the pediatric geneticist who sees kids. I wrote this letter, and I send photos of myself, and I send every reason why I think I have it. She calls me, and says I'll take your case! My Mom came up for Thanksgiving, and she came with me, which meant so much to me. We went and met Doctor Natasha Shur. She was so incredible! She was so happy, and excited, because she had never diagnosed someone my age. So, she's looking at me, and she said I have something with the eyes. I don't remember the words. It's a very long word. Something with the distance between the eyes. My head is in the tenth percentile, at 35 years old. My pinkie toes, the toenails never formed. It was another symptom, or it can be. I told her about my organization, and my impulsivity. No patience. What she told me was … I told her about my birth Mom. She said I don't know how, because as much as your birth Mom drank, how you ended up so well. The only thing she can think is because of my parents. She thanked them because they raised me in an incredible environment. Also she thinks I metabolized the alcohol very quickly when I was in utero. Which makes sense. I drink occasionally, but I have to watch. I can drink a lot, and I'm not affected by it. I have a high tolerance to alcohol. I know I do have tendencies, but I'm not an alcoholic. I could see myself headed that way if I didn't have the family support I do. I would be a disaster. If I was single, I would be at bars every night. I wouldn't know my boundaries. I attribute 95% of my success to my parents. They pushed me, and they kept me in a routine environment. I was in a loving environment! They treated me as if I was theirs, and I was! It made such a difference.

I have two little boys. I have a seven-and-a-half-year-old, and a three-year-old. I am married. That is where my impulsivity is an issue with that. I make decisions without even talking to him. I go on Amazon, and order this, and this, and this, because I think we need these things. I make appointments without consulting him. I don't slow down!

I have a wonderful marriage. It does have its ups and downs. He is my rock, and he is my external brain. He is always there when I get overwhelmed. He is very supportive. When my kids were younger, I would get frustrated, and overwhelmed. Occasionally now, if I am trying to do one thing, like make breakfast, and they ask where's my juice, or can you help me with this, or can you do a puzzle with me, I have problems. If they have more than one thing going on, I freak out. Two years ago, I went with my Mom to Lego Land in Florida. We ended up leaving early. I was miserable. There was too much stimulus at the amusement park. I didn't know which way the rides were. I can't read maps either. My son fell down. I yelled at my Mom. It was over nothing, but it was just too much! I get like that in situations where there are a lot of people, and a lot of things going on. I started seeing a cognitive-behavioral psychologist. The geneticist told me they help my impulsivity. So, what they told me to do, if I get overwhelmed, you have to stop. I close my eyes and take a break. I am tired all the time. I have always required a ton of sleep. I wonder if when I get stressed, I become exhausted. I have a prescription for B vitamins. It helps with energy. The counsellor I am seeing does something called "Mindfulness". We practice that, but it's hard. It's hard for anybody, because we are in such a fast-paced society. I adapt to change quite well. I don't think that my brain goes down deep enough to really be affected by that. Everything that hits me is kind of on the surface. If something changes, it can take me a while to get a hold of it, but I'm ok with it. I am a happy-go-lucky person. I love everybody.

Now, I wish I was given this diagnosis years ago. I am very immature. I am very smart, which I guess a lot of people with FASD are. But, I am immature socially. I prefer friends a lot younger than me, which is something that goes with FASD. I'm 35, but I love to hang out with the 21-22-year olds. So, my choices growing up, I was the perfect teenager. I was the perfect kid, until I reached 17 years of age. Then I dated a 35 year old. He was my track coach, and my substitute teacher. I tell everyone this story, because it's out there. I don't know why I did that. I don't know if that was part of the FASD. I don't know if it was part of my impulsivity. He ended up getting his license taken away. Emotionally, I was about 7 – 8 years old. I looked to him like a Father. I felt so very guilty, because I hid it from my parents. They found out, and they wanted me to stop seeing him. I did, but then he came around again, and I started seeing him again on the side. My parents found out again. It was a vicious cycle. I went off to college. We were still dating. Then one day, my college friends told me it was wrong. I ended it. I told him I needed to live life as a teenager. So, I ended it, with the help of the church. Back in college, I was involved in a Christian Group. Some people thought they were a little cult-ish. Not in a bad way. They slept together. They did everything together. They ate together. All the events, we went as one big group. They supported each other in every situation. I enjoyed it. But once I broke up with that guy, I decided I wanted to start drinking and have fun, so I stopped going. They weren't drinkers, and I wanted to drink on the weekends. I'm not involved in church anymore, although I want to be. I would like to take my kids, so they can learn, and then one day, they can make their own decisions.

I am proud of my two boys, because they're sweethearts. I am proud to be a Mother. Being a Mother is incredible to me. I am proud of the fact that I can do what my birth Mom was unable to. I don't blame her. I like to have fun, and I am a big kid at heart! I am proud because I have been able to be successful with school, with my job and as a woman who has her own family. I am very proud!

ADVICE - *Enjoy life and have fun. Not every day is going to be a bad day.*

CHAPTER 2
Kiera K.

Organization is a big thing with FASD!

I found out about FASD when I was diagnosed at the age of fourteen. That's when my Mom was like, ok! After all the years of testing through school and me struggling, and me struggling at home with home life, my Mom was finally made the appointment with the pediatrician and finally said like...ok! So I didn't know I was pregnant until I was about four and a half months. I went through the whole process and tests. I went through a two-day assessment, and that's when I was diagnosed with FASD.

For me, it didn't provide a lot of answers for me. I didn't think that there was anything wrong with me, personally. I thought that every kid struggled the same way I struggled. I had no idea! I had sensory disorders. I get overwhelmed. I thought every kid had that. If the lights were too bright, then their eyes hurt too. Or if sounds were too loud, then their ears would hurt too. It was normal to be….not able to sit still for long periods of time, or get distracted easily. I just thought that it was how every kid was! I didn't think I was different. I felt that I was somehow flawed in some aspect, because I was constantly being put through so much testing and had to do the specialized classes. But I didn't really understand why…..or you know? I did always have this sense of being flawed but not different. But at the same time, a lot of my difficulties were the same that other kids were struggling. I just thought that they could deal with them better. I didn't really understand. I think I chose not to understand….I'm not sure. I just accepted it, but I wasn't ok with it. I hated having to miss all the fun stuff because I was stuck in special ed class. I hated that I couldn't sit in the same class as everyone else the same way that they could. But I didn't really put all the puzzle pieces together. I don't know if I could put all the puzzle pieces together.

I didn't deal with my difficulties so well as I got to be an adult. It wasn't until I was about twenty-six is when I finally started to accept it all. I was angry throughout my childhood once I got my diagnosis, and once I started learning more about it. Mom took her career in the field. I resented her. I felt like why are you taking my struggles and sharing them with the world, and you're just trying to make yourself feel better for screwing me up. I was really angry, and I was really resentful. My sister and I had a really terrible relationship. We didn't get along, and she just had this....she was out to get me for some reason. I never really understood. So, I was a very angry child. I suffered with umm....depression and I had several suicide attempts starting at a young age. But I just never really put it all together up until I was about twenty-six. I finally agreed to get some therapy, and I went through two very serious suicide attempts before I was twenty-six and they were six months apart. Both attempts of suicide, I was using. I started when I was about twenty-four, I started abusing substances. I was never really a big drinker. I partied lots and I drank when I was about eighteen, and then I became a Mom at nineteen, so I never did party a lot. I missed out on that whole stage. Then I got divorced at twenty four, and my ex-husband had my kids, so that's when I kind of like....went back to the whole eighteen year old party kid. I began to drink heavily. It was a very difficult time. Those were kind of my wake-up calls...the suicide attempts. The first one was kind of when I went to the psychiatric center for three months. That was my first suicide attempt. That was in February. Then in August, I had another one that landed me on life support and I was put in a coma. When I came out of that, the doctor told my parents that this will be the rest of your daughter's life. And she is going to continue until she is successful. And that's when I was kind of like…mmmm! No! No, I don't think so! I started really researching FASD, and all of the secondary disabilities that come with it, and I went on the medication therapy, and I learned how to cope, and schedule, and how to function day to day. I learned to take things day to day, and that's when I decided that I was going to speak about FASD and change the stigma behind it that it's not all negative. I graduated from high school, and I graduated from college, and I was married, and I have two beautiful children. So now, I speak to people. I speak at adoption clinics, and it's not all doom and gloom when it comes to FASD. You just have to develop the proper coping skills, and proper therapies and help, get support for themselves, and then we can be successful with the proper encouragement and the proper education and everything like that.

I went through cognitive therapy as well as directorial behavioral therapy. I'm no longer in any therapies. Through the John Howard, we do the hall group which FASD action hall where it's an advocacy group. I co-facilitate that with Katarina. It's just teaching basic life skills, and how to deal with it in the workplace by saying "I have this disability. What I can do today, I might not be able to do tomorrow. Sometimes I may need a little extra time to do something." Just basically teaching people to be very open, and not be ashamed of their disability, because by being ashamed of it, and keeping it to ourselves, we're not helping ourselves. If we can verbalize that we have this disability, and what our strengths and weaknesses are, and where we may need a little extra help, it gives us a chance to be more successful in the workplace, and in the home, or any other aspect in life.

I recognize that I have come a long way. Some days, I'm like am I doing this for myself? Is this all in vain? Then I get emails, and letters from people who say "Your story is such an inspiration! You've given me hope that I can be somebody in life, and that I don't have to be the diagnosis…the label! That I can overcome those things!" If I can just help one person, then it makes this all worth it. But for me, it's just like, it was really hard to open up and share my story, because I have a really…..I don't want people to pity me. That's not why I do this! I don't want attention. I don't want people to pity me. I don't want people to feel sorry for me, because I don't feel sorry for myself. I don't pity myself. My life is what it was, and I've been able to overcome all of that. I have my own home. My kids are in my life. These are big things, and these are all things that people don't realize that we are capable of. So, I want to show other people who are still in that dark thought of being their disability…to show them that it doesn't have to be that! That you can step out of that being ashamed, because it's not something that we chose to have. Once people understand that it's not our own choice that we have this brain damage, then people are a little more accepting of it. It's no different than having any other disease, any other disability or any other….anything! We are good people if given the chance to be!

I'm divorced now. It was a good divorce. It needed to happen. It was…we were young, and it wasn't a very good relationship, but we just stayed good friends. He's re-married. He's doing much better. He was an alcoholic. He turned his life around. I am much better on my own. That's the thing that people don't realize with FASD! We ARE strong people! And for us to keep on keeping on every day, is huge! People don't understand that every day can be a big struggle for us. For us to keep going every day, is huge! People with FASD have to overcome so many adversities, so many challenges every day. They still get up the next day and keep going. People don't recognize that. People with FASD aren't given the credit where credit is due! This is why I do what I do! It's my passion! It's my goal! It's just something that is very important, and near and dear to my heart. You know, my Mom….she's an advocate for FASD. In the past year, when I started speaking, I would tell everybody…"No, I'm not angry at my Mom! My Mom didn't do this to hurt me." No mother, no matter what situation takes a bottle or puts a drink in their hand and says "My kid's not going to ever be able to read, or comprehend because….." No matter the situation, no mother intentionally means to harm their child that way. It's a lack of education. I was really bitter at my adoptive

Mom. I was like, "How could you take my disability and make it your career off of my struggles?" I have just realized in the past year that my Mom didn't do it to make herself feel better, or to gain from our struggles. She's about PREVENTING FASD, so that no family has to live the life we lived. In the past year, I have accepted that, and I called my Mom to tell her that I am not angry! I don't resent you anymore. I understand now why you do what you do. I understand that you didn't hurt me on purpose.

At the John Howard, we have general practitioner students who come in every week. In their medical texts books, there is only <u>one paragraph</u> on FASD….that's it! So, we have the students come in and sit in on one of our group sessions, so that they can see how we are, and how we act, and how we just are…..you know! Because a lot of times, we'll go into to our doctor, and they'll be like "Oh yah, whatever! You're just this…or you just want attention, or you just want pills, or you're just an addict. Or something! You're this! You're that!" We get dismissed as having anything wrong with us, when we don't really know what's wrong with us. It's because we have such a hard time verbalizing what exactly is wrong with us, and why we need help. So, we are kind of just written off. So, what I do is I also ….what I say at the John Howard, is to take a binder, and if you're diagnosed with anything, get a copy of it, and put it in your binder. So that when you do have to go into a walk-in clinic, you have the paper work showing that I have FASD, or I have degenerative disc disease. I have…..umm….stomach problems. I have all these mental health issues. I have the list of medications I am on and have been on for however many days. I have that documentation with me when I walk in. Going in to see a new doctor can be extremely overwhelming. So much so that we often end up shutting down. This way, when I tell them to put everything into a binder, I've taught them to bring those papers. And do this EVERY TIME you go to the doctors. Bring these papers with you whether it's your family doctor that you see regularly, or if you see any other doctor.   That way if you start to get overwhelmed, or you don't know what exactly to say, you can just say, "Here is my paperwork!"

People who have FASD are able to relate to me better than they can with anyone else. It's why my goal is to continue with the self-advocacy group. Because it's a safe place for us. It's where we can take our mask off. We don't have to be who society wants us to be. We can be open and honest. We encourage each other. We can relate to each other, and we can help each other... those who are battling these battles. We feel so alone. So when you have somebody else who you can say," Hey! I know exactly what you're talking about! That happened to me last week! How did you get through it, because I ended up shutting down and walking away!" Those peer support groups are key! When I first started at the John Howard, I had just started going to the group. We had people who wouldn't talk or open up. And I got a chance to share my life story at the group. And from there, all the other members of the group really started opening up and speaking...they were more comfortable sharing their life story, and their struggles. They finally had someone who had the same story! Someone that they could relate to. It was someone who they were like, "Well, you've overcome...then I can overcome, so I am going to come to you if I need advice and when I need someone to talk to." We're all very close. We all keep in contact. We all have each other's cell so that if there are any problems, and they need someone to talk to, we're there. A lot of professionals know all about it from books, but the real experts are the ones who live with it every day! The people who live with it every day….they know how it works. The professionals should sit down with those who know what it's like and ask us how we can help them. How we can gain from other people who live with FASD. That's what professionals should really do! But because we have the FASD label, nobody will give us the time of day for us to say what we need, and how it works for us.

On hard days, sometimes, I have to take it by one hour, one minute even. I just keep on keeping on. So, I know today might be a really bad day, but I don't know what tomorrow's going to bring. If I can make it through this really bad day, I'm facing a really good day tomorrow. We have two choices. We can sit down, lay down, cry, wallow in self-pity and say why me? Why me? But that's not going to get us anywhere. So, if you're having a bad day, sit down a cry. Have your moment, but get up and keep going, because tomorrow is a brand new day. Nobody else is going to feel bad for us, so if I'm having a really bad day, some days I need to sit down and cry! Some days, I just need to say ok! Enough is enough! I'm done for the day! I'm just going to relax! I'm going to shut down, but I know that I can't just continue to stay shut down. I got to keep going and figure out where I went wrong today. Maybe I woke up 10 minutes late. Ok! So, I'm going to set my alarm a little bit earlier tomorrow. You got to take it as it comes, learn from it, and adjust for the next day.

The best way for us is to stay in a routine. Sometimes I need a hand with that. In the past, what I've learned in the past two years is to reach out. I can call my Mom and be like "Look! I'm having problems with AISH. I need you to take over that for me, because I'm just...it's not working for me. So, can you make those calls for me?" When I reach out to Katarina at the John

Howard, I'm like, "Look! I'm really struggling! I don't know where to turn to get the resources I need. Can you help me?" and not be ashamed for asking for help. For years, I wouldn't ask for help from anybody. I was doing it on my own. I didn't need nobody's help. I didn't want nobody's help, and I was just going to do it. The biggest thing I ever learned…. it's no different than somebody who's in A.A., or who's an addict. Pick up the phone! It's ok to ask for help! It doesn't make us any less of a person if we need help, you know!

So, I have my binder which organizes my bank papers, my bill papers. It's like a file folder but in a binder, so I've got…I've got extra paper in there, cause I work on my presentation all the time. So, if I have a new idea, and I want to update my presentation, it's there, but I also have my original presentation. I have my…when I was working, my job description. My duties for work. If I was having a bad day, then I needed that as a reminder. All my medical information is in there. And I also have an agenda. I also have it in my purse, so that I can look at it every day, and I can know exactly what was going on, or I know what's happening for the next day, or tomorrow. If don't have it…if I forget to write it in my agenda….fooof!! I forget complete about it! So, it's just learning tools, and not being afraid to reach out, and ask for help when you're not sure. And then it makes life so much easier.

I moved from the Edmonton area to pursue my motivational speaking, and my FASD work which is why I moved here. My mom still lives up north. The Lakeland Centre up there is like the leading centres in all of Canada, and they have the very first ummmm…..women's only treatment centre for pregnant women. Where it's a live-in residence. It's called The Second Floor. It's for…it's a…it's a…. addictions rehab for women.

At the group, we focus on what other people's strengths are. We all draw from that…whatever their like…..so we may be able to one day help them build strength. My best friend also has FASD, and I met her at the International FASD breakfast in Calgary last year. Her Mom is big in the FASD community, as well. She is my best friend, and her weakness is my strength, and her strength is my weakness. We balance each other out. So, we both draw inspiration from each other. "I know you can do it! You've overcome it, so maybe I can too!" If she's having a bad day, she'll call me. I can get her calmed down, and we will problem solve together, and get it all worked out. If I'm in the same situation, I will call her be like "I don't know what to do!" She is really good with money, and stuff. Some days, I'm not! She'll come help me budget. She'll help me figure out that stuff. When it comes to problem solving, and scheduling, and like….my memory is stronger than her memory. She'll be like, "I don't know what's going on!" and I can be there to explain it to her. We really rely on each other.

ADVICE – don't ever give up! Every day is a new challenge, and as long as you keep going, then you'll be ok. You are who you are, and FASD doesn't define you as a person. You're so much more than just a label. Don't ever be ashamed of who you are and focus on your accomplishments and successes. Not your failures and mistakes. Everyone makes mistakes!

CHAPTER 3
Myles H.

I was adopted when I was around three or four years old. I'm Metis. My Mom was Cree. My Dad was French. I have about nine siblings in my biological family. In my adoptive family, there are eleven of us kids. And my adoptive parents are amazing. They have fostered over seventy kids, adopted nine of us, and have two of their own biological children. All nine adopted children have varying disabilities. There's four of us on the fetal alcohol spectrum. It was always entertaining growing up in a house full of kids! You didn't realize how busy it was, because it's normal to you when you grow up in it.

I grew up in Calgary. I was born and raised in Calgary. My parents were Mormon, and that was good because we had a lot of family time together. That came with routine and structure.

We always knew what the days were going to look like, and what was happening, so that was really key for me. Knowing what was happening. Going in to the school, I was really hyper, and a pretty happy kid. When I was adopted, my parents were told that I had at the time, FAE (Fetal Alcohol Effects). But they didn't really give much information on it. They just knew that my Mother drank while she was pregnant with me, and so back then it was, "He might have some learning disabilities." That's it!! That was the early '80's. There wasn't much information. The hard part was that, because if you didn't have those facial features of somebody with full-blown FASD, it was thought back then that you didn't necessarily need the same supports, and it was seen more as a learning disability. But because it wasn't talked about, and not much was known about FASD, it kind of turned into behavioral issues. And so behavior problems would jump to punishment. And so, from a young age, I was seen as…..not listening, not behaving. Then it turned into lazy. Now, I'm late for school all the time. That was around grade five, if not earlier, if I remember. I lived a block at the most, away from the school. I would come up the back alley, cross the street, and I'd be at the school. It wasn't like I lived far away. But that's where my struggles with getting to places on time started was around grade five. And so, my grade five, for me, that's where I really started to see those different labels being given to me. I saw that I was different from the other kids. I was weird and silly, and I would do odd things and then a couple of minutes after I did them, and I'm standing by myself, because everyone laughed and walked away, I would wonder…why did I do that? Why do I act like that? Why am I so weird and silly? So, uhh, you know, for myself, I didn't have answers. We just didn't know about FASD back then. My parents couldn't explain it to me. Even if they could, at that young age, it wouldn't make any sense.

School started to become a struggle at the end of elementary. Going into junior high, things seemed to get more intense. I began to have even bigger struggles, because now you have an even bigger school. Everything else has gone up. Expectations have all gone up. You have more information to learn. You have more people around you, which is more sensory stimulation. You have more rules. But it seems with all of this more stuff, you have less time. In elementary, I was in an L.D. class; a learning disabilities class. So, it was good in that I could take more time to do my work, and we had more teachers. So, there was about eight to twelve of us kids in that class, and two or three teachers. Now, going into junior high, it was now one teacher, and I was in the regular classes with thirty or more kids. So, I didn't have that one on one time. Didn't have the time to have the teacher come and explain things, and break it down, and then repeat it to me again. It was very easy to get lost in all of the stuff that was going on. But it was also easy to start to fade away, because it became.....OK! I won't put my hand up, and they won't know that I don't know how to do the work, and I can just sit here and just not do the work. So, those names, and those labels that I was given in elementary, I was starting to take on...partly intentionally in junior high. "Yeah, you're right! I am lazy! That's why I'm never here on time! Yeah, you're right! I don't care. That's why I didn't do the homework. Yeah, you're right! I'm not trying! That's why I don't know how to do this work in class." Because at that point, it was a lot easier to take those labels and name tags, than stand up and go "No! I'm too stupid! No, I'm dumb." I'm this, I'm that, or whatever it is. Whether it was those things that they were saying I was or, the names that I was giving myself. Me falling behind was beginning to put a strain on my Dad especially, because he was the one that we did the home work with all the time. So, he was the one that I fought with all the time. And, he would try to teach and to help, but the problem was that I couldn't remember how to do the work that I did at school when I was at home, because it had been however many hours. I can't remember how to do the work from twenty minutes ago sometimes, so how am I going to remember it hours later? So, my Dad would try. Then he would get frustrated, and I was coming home frustrated already. That's the thing, is that you need to understand is that coming home, you have already been kicked, and pushed down and you are done. You're done! You have no energy left. You have no motivation. You're just emotionally, mentally and physically done! So, to come home and do more of that stuff is not going to happen. So, there were the problems there. But also, in junior high, is where it started to have some physical issues, and there were time where my knees and my legs would be so sore, that I struggled with walking. I would go out, and would be fine, and then I would have to call my Dad and say, "Can you come pick me up?" I've got my bike, but my knees hurt too much to go any farther. So, my Dad was great. No questions asked. He always came and got me. There wasn't much thought or much hesitation to question me. Yeah, there wasn't much thought to look into the physical stuff at the time, and so I was struggling with my knees hurting, and struggling with something that would happen every once in a while. I couldn't sit or stand. It was quite painful. It would last for a few minutes. So, my Dad would take me to the hospital, and we saw the doctor, and they would say "You've got a hernia, but it's nothing big. Don't worry about it." This would continue to happen. So, we thought well, of course, doctor said don't worry about it. Ok, sure! So, it continued on. The learning problems were coming to be the main issue. Behavioral problems started to happen because of the troubles learning. You're told you're a bad kid in enough ways, you believe it, and you become that, right? I was a good person. My parents who adopted me have amazing hearts. Great people, and instilled in me the things that matter. Kindness, compassion. That's who I was at the core. But I was struggling, and I began rebelling. It was like, "Well, this is what you think I am! Ok! Fine! Sure!" I couldn't see any other reason why not. I was totally frustrated. I know in junior high, it was a matter of I was trying to get out of school, because this is where all the problems are. So, going to a place where you're a failure every day for eight hours, you don't want to go there. Why? Why do you get up every morning? Oh, I don't want to go there and bang my head against the wall, and be told how much of a failure I am. You get to the point where you just get out of school, and then we can get past all these problems. I made it to grade 11, and then I left school. I was told to leave, because I couldn't pay for the school bus.

It was the summer of going into grade eleven. At that point in my life, I had left home. I had met these guys who I thought were my friends and started to get into drugs and alcohol with them. It was the first time that there was that acceptance, and I didn't have it with any of my peers in school where I was accepted, because I was weird, and couldn't do this or that. So, here now, I was being accepted because I was doing drugs and alcohol. I couldn't be doing that while living at home because of the kids that my parents had. It was too dangerous because of the guys I was hanging out with to be having that stuff at my parents' house. So, they said I needed to leave. By that point, I was angry, and I was a mad teenager, and I knew everything! So, I was like fine! I don't want to be here anyways. So, I left home at seventeen years old. Now, I was chronologically seventeen, but functioning around about a fourteen-year-old. So, if you can imagine a fourteen-year-old doing drugs and alcohol and living on the streets. It's not going to go over so well! Things started to really spiral out of control. Days were filled with just drinking, and doing drugs. I started to get jobs, because I needed the money. I ended up having all the same problems that I had in school now start to be the same problems in my work. Work became a problem, because I couldn't keep a job. I had a lot of different jobs that I had for a few years. I could get them very easily, but I couldn't keep them. Again, all those names, and things that I had heard in school, I was hearing in the workplace. You're lazy! That's why I'm not showing up on time! I can't remember how to do the job! Again, whether it was someone saying it, or I was saying it to myself, at that point I was feeling really lost in life, and completely alone.

How did I know I was different? You see other people, and you see the steps that they're taking, and in school you see how their learning, and how they're getting all that stuff. It looks easy for them. You ask yourself, "Why don't I get all of that? Why can't I?" The brain doesn't work the same. It just doesn't make sense. I could see people taking those other steps and milestones, so, it was hard to understand why everyone else seemed to be moving forward, and taking those steps, and why not me?

I ended up finding my biological family. I was nineteen when I found them. At that point, I was lost, alone and struggling so much that that was going to be the thing that was going to change everything for me. Looking, believing and moving forward to find that thing that was going to make that change in life. Cause this isn't how you live life. Nobody has this many struggles in life. Nobody suffers this much! Nobody has to go through all of this. There has got to be a change! When I ended up finding my biological family, I thought that that would be the good turn in my life. It ended up being one of the worst experiences of my life! I got the information from the adoption agency. "Here's your family!" They give that much to you. But they never tell you that it may never be that great, happy rainbow and fun times that you have pictured in your head, and that you've had pictured in your head for sixteen or seventeen years. I ended up finding out that both of my parents had passed away. My brothers were addicts who were living on the streets. What I thought was four or five of us in the family ended up being nine of us kids. We didn't know about each other. We grew up in other families. When we came together, it just didn't work out at all. I went into this world where I was now being used and abused by my family; my brothers, and sisters. I was being used and abused by my "friends". At that point, because I was feeling distant from my adopted family, didn't have a biological family that I had hoped for, I didn't have friends, I couldn't keep a job....I had nothing. Everybody has a purpose. I had nothing. That was a hard part to feel so completely alone and to have nothing. But there was always something inside me that was like "Keep going! Keep going!" I always thought that there had to be something, right? There's got to be something bigger. There's just got to be some better, and there has to be a purpose for me! I grew up like this, and I don't go to church, but I have my own relationship with the Higher Power. There's those times that you have to. When you're out there by yourself, on the streets, there's days when you got to give it up and be like, "Ok! I am giving it up to you! I can't do this!" It helps! If not, you are done. There are days when I would have been done, had it not been for my faith.

A lot of things that gets lost with FASD, are the secondary effects. The forgotten about effects. When you look at a child, the direction of their life starts to take place between the ages of birth to about three to five years of age. So, if you look at children's lives, and talking to individuals with FASD, you'll hear a lot of similar stories. It will be about the struggles in school, and them turning to addictions, and becoming homeless, and then getting involved with criminal justice. There are all of those similarities. What we don't realize is and understand is what happened before you were three, or what happened before you were five. If you're in an environment where there's a lot of abuse, drugs, or alcohol, and you're not getting the things that you need. Nutrition, housing, clothing…all of those things, that plays a huge role in your life. As great as my parents were who adopted me, and couldn't have loved me anymore, I had already been set on this path where things were affecting me. I had attachment disorder. Before I was adopted, I went through seven or eight different foster homes. When I was a little older, I thought if they loved me, they would have kept me. Those things that you start to experience as you get older and see more have had an impact on your whole life. It's those secondary things that play a huge role.

You have these problems with FASD. You have problems with reading, and writing. You maybe look a certain way. But what you don't realize is that this is something that I didn't find out until my very early years of getting into learning about FASD was when I met Liz. She talked about FASD, the full body diagnosis. That was the first time that I had heard anybody talk about the physical parts. Going back to my youth, I had been working odd jobs for the longest time. I met this lady, Liz, at the job I was working at the leisure centre. We became friends. She shared with me that she was doing a conference on

FASD. She invited me to come and speak at the conference. So, I went to the conference, and I spoke at it. After I was done speaking, it was this "A-ha!" moment. I was absolutely in a dream! It was my realization of, "This is it!!" I wasn't sure what "it" was, but it was like yeah! There's something here! That started with someone else coming up to me and telling me they're were having a conference in Edmonton. It just went from there. I continued to go around public speaking. At one that was being held in Calgary, Liz was there. She was talking about parts of the body being affected, and this being what FASD looks like. As she was going through the list that she had, I was sitting there going "Yup! Yup! Yup!!" That for me is where I tell people I got my diagnosis. That's where FASD made sense! I was able to understand and realize that I'm not lazy and so on. I struggle with sleeping, so I can't function like everybody else. I never sleep! So, this began to make sense! I have this thing I call "bubble trouble". Imagine thousands of bubbles in your body. I can't sit still. When I go home at night, there's no off switch before I go to bed. My brain is constantly firing, and because my sensory issues are so high, everything else around me throughout the day is still happening. Clothing feels. That smell. That lighting. That sound! When I go home at night, I would try to go to sleep, but I can't because of that buzzing of the fan was still grabbing my attention. The wind blowing. The way the sheet felt on me. All of these things get noticed by me. So, I never slept! I didn't realize this for thirty odd years…. thirty-three I think I was when I was finally able to go to the doctor to get some medication to help me sleep. I began to learn so much about myself, and how to take care of my body. I have to take B12 vitamins, and it helps with energy. Liz taught me about what she called the full body diagnosis. The full body diagnosis talks about the bones, and the muscles, and how alcohol affects those things being developed. Those times that I was struggling as a young kid with walking and having sore joints and stuff like that go along with the FASD. Years later, when I got the physical diagnosis with my FASD, that's where I got to understand the health issues. Over the last three or four years, Liz and I have been going to the doctor and getting stuff done and that's where we found hip dysplasia, scoliosis, osteoarthritis in my ankles, my knees, elbows. I have degenerative aging disease in my neck. All of this stuff, and I am only 37! I exercise a lot, which help to open up my hips and joints.

I started doing the motivational speaking, I was mentored by her, and I learned many things from her. I started attending these conferences where I began speaking. I started going to the sessions. It became important for me to understand FASD. I want to and need to understand myself! In that realization and understanding of FASD came acceptance.   There were reasons and there's answers behind how I was now. REAL reasons, and those honest answers to what's going on instead of putting those name tags and labels on them! I wasn't broken on purpose! That was so important for me! This all began about ten years ago when I started working at different agencies running mentoring groups. It was great, because as I was doing this, I was starting to see the similarities that I had with other individuals. I could relate! This was good, because I could share my experiences, and they would share theirs. Even though they weren't always the same, or we didn't feel the same about it, it was always nice to know that someone else is going through that, or has been that. It was huge! I felt understood. As much as I was helping them, it was helping me. It drove me more to want to do it for other people who were struggling. I found that I was able to see where I had been through these things, and now I had found my reason for going through all of that. My reason was so now I can help all of these other individuals! The ones that are living on the streets or in the park, who are being taken advantage of by their "friends". I can say I get it! You know that they're not your friends, you sometimes know that they're using and abusing you, but how do you walk away from it when you have nobody else? The group I hung out with used to only hang out with me if I had money. One day, I got beat up pretty badly by my "friends". I should have walked away, but after I got a bit better, who did I go back to visit? The same people who beat me up. Another example, if you get a new place to rent, and you get set up with that, it's not like when they give you the new place that you'll also get a new, good, healthy group of friends. So, you get the new place, but who do you invite over to celebrate your new place? Those guys that lived in the park with you. They come, they get drunk, and do drugs. They don't care! They smash the place up, and what do they care? Who deals with the consequences? Who ends up getting kicked out, and has to find another place? I had trouble understanding the cause and effect of everything. Whether it was fighting in elementary school, and then standing there when the kid ran away, and the teachers would come over. I would be like "What? We got into a fight because he started it! Why would I run away?" That little brain inside, or the voice that everyone else had that said, "This is a bad thing! Run away, so you don't get caught!" I didn't seem to have that. I pulled a fire alarm, and everyone ran away while I stood there. There were three friends around me. It was a dare. I was like ok, and I did it. Reasons being were:

a. Because I was dared. I want to look good.

b. This was the biggest thing. Every day I would walk past this little red box that said, "DO NOT PULL."

I knew it made this sound. My sensory issues were like, "WHOAAA!" I have an inability to control my impulses and maintain that because it's like I HAVE to do it! People don't understand that that not giving into impulsivity can physically hurt, to the point where it's like "Ow! Ow! Ow!" I can't handle it physically. It's not that I wouldn't like to. It's just that I physically can't. It is physically uncomfortable, and so you do it even thought you know you're not supposed to, you're like, "Ahh! I did it!" It's like a reward. Meanwhile, everyone else reacted, and inside it was a relief.

In junior high, while working during the mentoring program, there's this bell at the receptionist desk, and all the young adults that came in for the mentoring group hit that bell. "Ding! Ding! Ding!" I'm like, "K, guys! We can't do that" And then they would tell us, "Ok! You have to tell your kids that not to do that!"

The problem was… I wanted to do it too! Why? Because of that "ding" and it was like, "Ahh!" It's there, so it's like "Hey!" No one else sees it, no one else feels it. To manage that impulse to make the bell "ding", I ended up putting it under the desk. Actually, I ended up taking it home!! Still the issue was I still knew where it was. I could reach under the desk, and make it ding. It's a matter of if I feel that, can I change that feeling? As I have gotten older, I have become more self-aware. This has all helped me so much to help me understand FASD, to explain things, and to make sense of it. With my "bubble trouble", I actually have my audience blow bubbles, so they can understand the reasons for moving. You can't make it stop. It helps me with my own self-awareness. I still get that need to react to it but do it in a way that is socially acceptable. You can't just say, "Don't!" You can't! It's just not there in us. You have to find coping mechanisms. If someone says "don't" to something, like don't touch the cookies! For us, it's like, "Well, I wouldn't have if you didn't say anything!!" The fact that it has been pointed out, now I have to! Impulse control can be a problem for people who have FASD.

When I was seventeen, I mentioned I was functioning around the age of a fourteen year old. I was hanging around guys who were carrying weapons, stealing cars, breaking into houses, dealing drugs. It was a rough neighborhood I grew up in. It was hard for me because I would rather talk about what I saw on Sesame Street that day, but I couldn't because it could get me into a situation. I couldn't be this funny, silly guy with those hard core guys that I was hanging out with. It was a struggle. Sometimes, I couldn't control it. However, we'd be at a party, and because there was drinking and drugs, I could pass it off as being drunk. I was very dysmature. It was hard when I had to be cool, and an adult, because I couldn't be me. Looking back, when we were partying, do you think we were eating? No! We were just partying. Also, looking back, I highly doubt that I was the only one on the spectrum! I actually ran into a couple of my old friends over the past couple of years. Some of them are still struggling in that world still. One of them that I do remember well, he ended up passing away. He grew up in that hard environment, lived in it, and never got out of it. I haven't' seen too many that have been able to get out. It's unfortunate. You have to do it for yourself.

Since getting to know Liz, and working as a motivational speaker, I have become quite well known in the FASD community. I heard about all of the bad stuff about FASD. We won't get to finish school. We won't be able to get a job. If we do get a job, we won't be able to keep it. You know! I wanted to share the positive stuff, so that people don't just look at the bad things. That is what my story always was. Here's my story. Here's my struggles. Here's the issue. Here's the growth, and here's where we are now. It was routine and repetition. It was an acceptance of myself because I learned about FASD. How do I live my life? I live it through that understanding. You take what you went through, and you try to learn from it. There is a purpose. I wanted to get that message out there. When I am in a conference, I ask the audience, if you can relate to any of these things that I am talking about, please stand up. By the end of that, almost everyone would be standing up, because everybody has struggles. Money management issues, self-esteem issues, addiction issues. All of these issues. Whatever it is, all of those things that I speak of are package of the things that I experience. It all made me who I am. People are surprised when they can relate to that.

In all of my presentations, I share that you can become a victim of FASD, or you can become resilient. Victim who suffers from FASD….that was a headline that was put in the news after I did an interview about FASD, and introduced the Minister of Children's Services who was coming in to introduce the ten year strategic plan. It was a huge honor! I was super excited! Very nervous! I did it and it went great! Did all of these interviews with newspapers, and Liz helped me out. While Liz and I were out one day, I saw a paper, and it had that headline. All I saw was "victim" and "suffers." I asked Liz, "Really? Is that all they got out of it?" We hear that all the time. But I don't' suffer. It is NOT who I am, because it doesn't define me. There is a big difference. I live successfully with FASD, and that is where the switch has to be. Most of the time, you'll find that people who have FASD have a big heart. That's how they survive and push through all of this stuff that you have to go through. You've got to be stronger than other people. You've got to have that heart, and that determination. Sometimes that looks like they have attitude, and that they always have to fight.

I have struggled with the agencies that I worked with, because even though I was a mentor and I was to work there speaking to people, I wasn't getting to work on time. I wasn't able to remember to fill out my time sheet. These are agencies that are known all over Canada, and agencies that work with kids and families with disabilities. You have an individual who has this one disability, and helping to run a program, yet that is the problem that I've run into. I have worked with agencies such as the John Howard Society and have had pre-med students come in to learn about FASD, because it is something that they don't know about. In their manuals, and textbooks, when I ask them about the information in them, they said that there is about a half a page of information about FASD in the entire text book. This has to change! Even now, when I go to conferences and talk about it and that it is a full body diagnosis, there are still people who are like, "What? I didn't know that!" It's still common. I'm glad that there are still people that I can help understand this.

There are days when it's busy, and I am thinking how I would love a day when I wasn't so tired. Or I would love a day when my bones don't hurt. Or I would love a day when everything is good. It's hard to have those days, because you wonder what's tomorrow going to be like. But through it all, I always remember to push through. I am so blessed to have the life I have. I have an amazing place. I am a full time motivational speaker, and I get to set my own schedule. I help with training. I am aware that I won't do good with anything unless it's in the afternoon. So, I set up appointments for the afternoon. I always joke at conferences that I speak at about time. We do well if it is later in the day. So, you have all of these people who have FASD who are supposed to speak at 8:30 in the morning…..you think that the conference would be set up for the afternoon! I have learned that early in the morning is hard for me. I set up for success, and make things happen later in the day, so I don't let anyone down. I still need supports. For me to be successful, I do have reminders. I will ask Liz to call me and remind me to check this email, or make this phone call. She is one of my external brains. Sometimes, people see me do things, and they forget that I forget how to do things. I have a schedule and routine set up so that I don't forget to pay my bills, or forget to buy groceries. Sometimes, I even have some reminders to eat! I rely on outside supports. I still have those days when things aren't great. I need people around me to be supportive. I need people to be loving and gentle with me. I have a great heart, and I care about people, so I try to surround myself with people who are the same, and who understand. Don't focus on the negative, and give it power. Always focus on your can do! Now, I have a good relationship with my adoptive parents. Looking back, they now understand. My parents tried to support me, they would see their little boy struggling, but with the lack of information about what I live with, it was hard for them. They didn't always know what to do. I always knew at the end of the day that they loved me. Even when we weren't getting along very well, I knew that they loved me. They didn't know it then, but they did the right things. Now, we celebrate this all together, because what I am now, and my motivational speaking, I wouldn't be here without them. So, this is all about our successes as a family.

ADVICE - *I need people around me to be gentle. I need people around me to be understanding.*

One thing that I have learned from my parents is to focus on the ability. Not the disability. So, that is where my focus is. The things that I struggle with, I just ask for help. It's ok to ask for help. Why not? That's how you can be successful.

CHAPTER 4
Joni R.

My name is Joni. I have lived in Calgary my whole life. I was adopted as a baby. I am Blackfoot. My adoptive Mom is Irish, and my Dad is English. I have had FASD since I was born, but I think I learned about it when I was around grade three or four. I started to realize that I was different, and I realized I couldn't run as well. My Mom taught me that I had heart problems which were contributing. That's when I started to learn about it. I was adopted. I had a good upbringing. I had a Christian upbringing. I wasn't always the kid who would get up and make my bed, or go brush my teeth. My parents were always telling me to make the bed or brush my teeth. Or it would be "Joni, why didn't you make your bed? Why didn't you brush your teeth?" Then they would tell me if I couldn't get up and make the bed or brush my teeth, I would never be able to get a job, or live on my own. But once I moved out, I wanted to prove to my Mom that I can do this! I'm going to prove to her that I can do everything that she says I couldn't do! Now, you know, she's totally changed her tune! She's like, "Joni, I'm so proud of you and of everything that you've been able to do!" She's blown away by everything that I have managed to do with my life. I graduated from school and finished grade twelve. My parents said they were going to push me as far as I could go. I managed to go all the way! I did have an aid in grade eleven and twelve. Without that, I never would have made it. I just didn't really care about school. I was like, I'm not going to really do anything with my life, so what's the point in even trying? I was getting ready to graduate, and I was listening to all of my friends talk about going to school, and that they would get a job, and raise a family. You know, I'm going to do this! I'm going to do that! The stuff that isn't that unusual to talk about when they graduate. I had no idea what I was going to do with my life. I felt like they were supposed to tell me, because I didn't think I would have a life beyond my parents because they were very protective of me. I felt like I would be tied to my parents for the rest of my life. I did live with them for several years after school. They were trying to find me a home. My aunt told me years later what happened at that time. She said that they were trying to find me a home, and she had cancer at the time. I was getting a bit aggressive because everyone said I was bored out of my mind. I had nothing to do other than sitting at home, and daydreaming about something. My daydreaming is my way of releasing energy. I would go out to breakfast with my parents too. I just wasn't really doing too much. I did end up getting aggressive with my Mom. I ended up pushing her, and I pushed her down the stairs. Not good stuff. The other family were telling my Mom that she needed to find me somewhere else to live, because they were scared that I would really hurt her. My Mom didn't have the heart to put me out. They started praying, and they finally got the answer they needed. She said that they could send me to Peter Lougheed Institutional Ward. So, I went there, and then I was there for a couple of months. Then they found me a home, which is the home I'm in now. I have been here for about eight years now. I moved here in 2007. I love it here! I call the manager here Jane my Aunty Jane. That's how close I am to her. She calls me her niece.

I don't know many people with FASD. If I do, then they have never actually said that they have FASD.

Since I moved out, things that have changed in my life are learning more about FASD. I also started volunteering. My Mom came to visit me, and she said that she was proud of me, so it made me want to keep doing this! When I moved to the group home, I was still wanting to prove my independence, so I tried to become a writer. I did end up finishing writing a book, but I never got it published. No one thought that it was really worth anything. I was proud of myself for completing the book. My book is about my characters. I discovered that I was artistic when I went on a medication when I was in grade 6. It helped me focus, and I just started drawing. I have been drawing ever since. The medication was life changing. Before the meds, all I could do was scribble! I have ADHD, autism, and FASD. I did have to stop taking the medication when I first moved into the group home, because they said it was affecting my heart. But I have still been able to draw really well! My characters are punctuation marks. I was in grade nine, and in English class we were learning about punctuation. Since grade eight, I had been reading about how Garfield was created, and I was thinking I could do something like that. In our class, we were divided into groups for a project. I was given the job of designing the map for our group. While I was designing it, I got the inspiration to turn the punctuation marks into characters! The reason why I decided to do that was because nobody had ever done that, and it was unique, which was exactly what I wanted. The question mark is actually a dog! I wanted to have a twist on it that no one had ever done! I sat in church one Sunday, and I began designing these characters. I asked myself how I would turn a question mark into a person. I placed an eye here, an ear here, a tail here and before you knew it, I had this character. I called him Question. I thought the name fit him perfectly. I would love to show you a picture of my characters. I was able to have my work published in a couple of books. One of my nephews helped me. I have been trying to make a book out of my comics for a while. It costs too much to do it myself. My nephew helped me get it printed. I published a second book last November. I published the book myself. A lot of people have seen my work. When I finish something, I try to make it look as professional as possible. I draw my comics on the computer now, with a tablet. I put them all together on a USB stick, and then I take them to a publisher, and he publishes them in a book for me. I do charge a price for my books. My first book, I gave them away for a donation. I knew that I would need to get the word out there. This is what I do to keep busy, and this is the business that I run. I am always looking for opportunities to expand. I have an email, too: punctassoc@hotmail.com. That's my business email. I have never had any training on how to run a business. I taught myself. I had some help but I just make some choices, and go with it. I know that there are a lot of people who don't know how to do that!

ADVICE - *To people who are struggling with FASD, my advice to you is to never give up. You never know what's around the next corner. Back then, I never knew that I would be successful, but I put my mind to it, and I achieved it. This is what I am going to do, and I am going to prove to everyone that I can do it. Everyone is shocked at how far I have come. Everyone is proud of me, and no one ever dreamed I would be here now. Some people need a little bit of independence. Parents need to believe in their kids. We do!*

CHAPTER 5
Kelly M.

I found out I had FASD seven years ago. I was adopted when I was six, but I had been adopted when I was three years old and sent back after six months. I think my Mom was my fifth family. So, my biological Mom tried keeping me, and then it said in the papers that she couldn't afford to keep me, so she put me with friends. She took me back, and couldn't afford to keep me, so she gave me to Children's Aid, and then finally it said I was covered in bruises, and I was one and a half or something. They think her boyfriend......I screamed every time a guy would come into the room. I would start screaming, so.....the Children's Aid just took me for the last time from her when I was one and a half. And then, ummmm, I was in a couple of foster homes that weren't very bad. And umm, yeah, I got adopted when I was three, and I didn't get along with the other little girl that they had. I was supposed to kind of be like a play mate, and I think I was trying to get the Dad's attention all the time or something…I don't know. So, they sent me back, and then my parents adopted me when I was six.

I was adopted in Toronto. So, they got me when I was six, and by the time I was eight, they had sent me away to a training school for a year and a half. Ummm! It was awful! It was a private school in London, Ontario. Because of my FASD, I would do stuff …they didn't know, right? So, they'd say go to school when I was seven, and was supposed to be going to school, but somebody would find me on the neighbor's roof, or in somebody's backyard playing with their swing set or places I wasn't supposed to be. So, they thought I was bad, bad, bad. I was disruptive in class, and ummm, so they sent me to that training school for a year and a half. It was in another city. It was in London, and I would take the train by myself. Like a two-hour train ride by myself when I was eight. Looking back, we all say "Oh my God!" Cause my twelve year old isn't even allowed to go to the store by himself! On that train, back then, you could go out on the very last car, and you could go out on a little porch, so you were actually outside the train. It was like a little balcony, and I remember going out there, and trying to see, and I would stick my leg out, and see if I could fly like Superman! Geez! The school was really bad. I was always being punished. I had to go there, because I left my coat on the train. One of my winter coats. I was always losing stuff! And I left a brand-new coat on the train and they made me go get rags at the Goodwill to wear. It was like and old lady's coat. And then two sets of really ugly clothes, so that was all I was allowed to wear. At night, I would have to wash one outfit, and then wear the other. All the kids would laugh

87

at me at school. I had to wash walls, and scrub floors to earn my coat back. There were boys in there, and if I did something wrong, I would have to stand in the corner, with my hands on my head. I remember I was wearing like a nightie. I had to go to the washroom, and they wouldn't let me go to the washroom, and I accidentally peed on the floor. The guys got it just like we girls did. We had to stand in the corner until I puked, or sleep behind the couch. It was nasty. My Mom that I have now isn't the same Mom that I had back then. She was totally different. She is much stronger now and will fight like a tiger if she has to. I asked her just a couple of weeks ago. Me and her were talking, and I just started crying. We were talking, and we usually don't talk about stuff like that, but it just happened to come up out of the blue. And then I was crying, and I said, "Did you know it was hurting me, Mom, or did you not know?" She just thought that they were the professionals, and they knew the best. Still, like, my son, when they tried….he goes to Hull, and when they are unfair to him, I'm all over them. Maybe because of the way I was brought up….I have three kids, and if I think that someone is doing something wrong, I had no problems standing up to them.

I went to that training school for a year and half. I was ten when I stopped. We moved to England for a year after I went to that school. That was even worse, because my Mom got pregnant with my sister. She was in a strange country, pregnant and with a daughter that nobody can understand. Over there, they are even more strict. So, the teachers were hard on me there! The teacher complained to my Mom, and it was really hard on her. After that, we were in Holland for a little while. And then we came back to Sarnia, Ontario when I was eleven years old. I had a pretty lonely childhood. My Dad was the kind of guy who just didn't want to deal with it. I didn't have a good relationship with him. He was really responsible! Like my Dad was the ombudsman for Shell. He always had a really good job, and everything, but he didn't really have time with us kids. He never had time to play with us. He was a very, very good provider.

Then high school time rolled around eventually, and it was just a nightmare, of course! By then, I was hanging around with older people, and uh....I didn't fit in with the good kids that were smart, and never got in trouble. At all! I tried! It didn't work, because I always wanted to make my Mom happy. I would try, but it didn't work. I would just say the wrong thing, or do the wrong thing. Do stupid things. And uh, so then I started hanging out with a tougher crowd. And ummm, yeah! I asked Mom why my she never home schooled me. She was so busy, and she was pregnant with my sister. She was also working on her degree. She didn't have time to home school me.

I had my first job when I was twelve. And I had a job in a candy store. I loved candy! I would eat so much sugar. To make a long story short, the store owner guy raped me. His house was attached to the variety store, and he was East Indian. His wife and kids were in another room in the house, and he brought out beers, and I didn't know like what was going on. Then he was like, "Have a beer! Have a beer!" He kept forcing beer on me. Meanwhile, the store's open, and I didn't know what to do. He started bringing out dirty magazines, and he wound up raping me. At the time, I was in a different school because I had been kicked out of all of the other schools. It was a school with only like six students, and we each had a desk. I told my teacher, because after school I was supposed to go to work, and I was sitting on the curb, and I didn't know what to do.

I explained why I wasn't going to work. I begged him not to tell anybody, but he told my parents. That was one of my bad experiences. It was the first time I had been sexually abused

So, I was hanging out with the wrong crowds, and I was still getting into trouble and everything, and ummm…I was skipping school all the time, and going hanging out, and getting kicked out of school all the time. Like all the time! I think I got kicked out of every high school that I went to for doing stupid things. After my parents adopted me, we moved to Sarnia right away when I was little. When I was thirteen, that is when I started doing drug, and snuck out my window late at night to go to the arcade, and stuff like that. Because I fit in perfectly with those bad kids. Even though I hated drugs the first time I did them, I couldn't stand it, but if I was to be accepted in those crowds, you have to. So, I started doing drugs at a young age, but I hated it, because I hated how it made me feel. I kept running away all the time, because home…..I was thirteen. There was a highway by my house. I would just jump in it, and I would stick out my thumb. Where ever I would go, I would go. When I started hitch hiking down to Toronto, I got raped a lot. It was really unsafe. When I turned sixteen, I moved out for good. I never moved back home. I moved into a biker club house in Kitchener with a friend. Satan's Choice club house. It was an awful experience. I asked my parents if I could come back, but they said no. Living in the club house, it was drugs all the time, and a place to crash. I didn't have to work when I was living there. I was living with a bunch of people who were lost like me. There were a lot of other people there. Three of us lived in a small attic. Then there was the main floor was the club house, and there was always bikers in and out. This went on for about a year or so, and then I met a guy. I got pregnant, and so I quit drugs, and drinking and everything. I moved into a house where you go when you're pregnant. I forget the name of it, but it was in Kitchener, and it was all pregnant teens. We were really looking forward to having the baby, even though I was turning seventeen. Shortly after an ultra sound, I lost the baby. Then I had to leave that home. So, I was pretty devastated about that. After leaving that place, I tried to live in a group home. I wanted to do good! The group home didn't last for very long, because you had to go to school to live there. You had to do good in school, and me and a friend were horsing around, and she dared us to run across to the park when we weren't supposed to go out at night. She told us to run across to the park, and come back, and she would let us in through the front door....but she didn't! She locked us out. We had to call them, and we were kicked out. I was very gullible! The other kids that lived there got me into trouble! It's kind of funny now. I eventually learned that people aren't always able to be trusted!

I met another guy, who is my kids' Dad. He was a drug dealer, and was quite a bit older than I was at that time. He dealt speed. It was through his influence that I started doing needles, and started doing hard drugs. It was really bad! I was walking around at ninety pounds, and I am five foot eight. I was getting thrown in jail all the time for possession. I was never picked up for crimes against people. I have a pardon now. Other times, I was picked up and put in jail for theft, or if my boyfriend was arrested, I would be out in the court house parking lot, and would break into cars to try to have enough money to bail him out. It was stupid things! I got pregnant when I was nineteen years old. At this point in my life, I had become a hard core drug addict. When I found out I was pregnant, I quit using. I ended up having a baby boy, and I was trying to raise him.

I don't know how! When he was one and a half, I got pregnant with my daughter. I was clean! I was twenty years old. Both of my kids are doing well, and are grown up. I am so proud of them!! They are my pride and joy!

When my daughter was just a baby, I started using again. At this point, I had split up with my kids' Dad. I went to rehab to get clean, but I wasn't successful completing the program. I had shared with the counselors that I had possibly been exposed to AIDS. At that time, AIDS wasn't understood, and because of the fear of AIDS because it was still a new disease, I was asked to leave. I remember they threw everything out of the fridge, they were cleaning everything, and put all the dishes through the dishwasher. They didn't know anything about AIDS back then. On my own, I was able to quit drugs, I had both of my kids, and wanted to move. My parents lived in Burlington at the time. I was able to move into a shelter in Burlington that my Mom helped me with. When I was in the shelter, I met a girl who said that we could go out, and the shelter would help look after the kids. I didn't know the city that I was in, so she took me around. We ended up at a crack house. I didn't use, and I was worried about my kids, so I called the shelter, and they told me that I had to be back by 11pm. I couldn't leave though, because this girl I went with was using crack, and was really high, and she just kept using more. I didn't know how to get back. The shelter ended up calling the kids' Dad to come and get them. Again, this was me trusting someone, and it ended up being bad for me. I expected to be going out for coffee, and it ended up being bad.

I went back to London. My ex had my kids for four years, and in that time, I got into the drugs really heavy. I still went to go see the kids. He would have his parents look after the kids, and she was the best woman with my kids! We still have a good relationship now! To this day, my ex and I still get along. It was tough that the kids weren't living with me, but I could see them whenever I wanted. Children's Aid wasn't involved, and it was a good situation for everyone.

The drug use left me overdosing thirteen times. My heart stopped, and I was brought back. To support my drug use, I worked as a stripper for years. I have been in a lot of dangerous situations. I was stabbed through the lung on two different occasions. The same lung! I was still doing stupid stuff. One time, my friend and I stole a cab. I didn't know how to drive, but she did. We knew the guy who owned the cab, and he was passed out drunk, so we took his keys, and we drove around the city London picking up fares! We had picked up a couple of guys who needed to go to St. Thomas. We were going way too fast!

The highway went from two lanes to one lane ad we had to cross a narrow bridge. My friend didn't know this area, and was driving way too fast. We had the choice of trying to go off the bridge, or go down the cliff, and she went down the cliff! We rolled the car, and the car accident left me with a broken neck. I had to wear a neck and body brace. I was in the hospital in my hospital gown, I got arrested. I had been in the hospital for a while, and the doctor probably gave the ok that I could be arrested. From the hospital to jail! I had to stay there for a little while. The details of everything get a bit fuzzy, but I remember doing what I had to do to survive. I hooked up with a guy who stole professionally. I was pretty when I was younger, so being supported by guys who could take care of me was easy. I lived this fast life until I was twenty seven. At the age of twenty seven, I cleaned my life up. I went to rehab to get clean. I got my kids back. I went back to school, and I met with a lady there who everyone said was a hard ass. To me, she was so gentle, and understanding. She was really kind, and she would remind me of things that I would forget to do. I didn't see the hard ass lady that everyone told me about. I just loved her! How it all started was when I was in jail, my Mom said when I wanted to go to rehab, I'll help you. She wrote me letters for years! Every month, my Mom would write me a letter. And it would follow me, and I would get it eventually! She kept that connection! She even wrote a book about all of the letters she sent me.

I was in jail one time, and I was looking out the window, and there was this little bird, and he was on the fence. I was thinking, "You're in jail just like me, buddy!" He flew away, and then I made a decision I will never go back to jail again! I want to be free like that bird! I told my Mom, and she came. The funny thing is, I had a guy waiting for me on a Harley, and here's my Mom!

She butts right in front of him, and she's wearing this big ol' flower dress! She plops herself down on the lawn! When you're getting out, there are people who are out there waiting for you right there. My Mom had become a strong willed woman, and she was determined to come and get her daughter. She didn't want to lose me. So, she butted in front of my buddy, and when I got out, she just grabbed me, and hustled me to her car! Isn't that awesome???? I never went back! I'm forty nine, and I never went back to jail!

I was twenty seven!! She drove me straight up to my Grandma's, because she knew that I would never even swear in front of my Grandma! I love my Grandma! I respect her. So, she took me up there, and meanwhile, she's making calls everywhere trying to get me in somewhere. But everywhere said that I would have to call them. But I wouldn't do it, because I have a fear of the phone! It's ok if someone calls me, I'm fine. But

I can't call someone else. To this day, my Mom makes most of my phone calls like that. My son is the exact same!

There was one place that agreed to take me, but it was in Windsor. It was called the House of Sophrosyne. It means balance. So, my Mom drove me from my Grandma's, which was like seven hours. She kept me at my Grandma's until it was time to go, and then she drove me there. She got me everything that I would need, because all of my other stuff was at a drug house. I said, "I gotta go get my stuff, Mom!" and she said, "The hell you are!" She bought me all new stuff. She drove me to rehab, and I stayed there for a month. They talked me into staying another month. Sharon, the lady who everyone said was mean, and who nobody like, was great! I just loved her. Every time that it was time for me to leave, they would tell me they thought I should stay. So, I would stay for another month. So, I stayed for three months, and then my Mom and Dad came down to Windsor, and got me a room. We didn't know the city at all, and they just got me a room. It turned out it was in a crack house. There was smoke coming through my vents, but it didn't matter. I hitch hiked in blizzards to get to meetings. I did good, because I didn't relapse. Then my kids came. I would take the bus to go see my kids at their Grandma's. She'd let me stay there for the weekend. I used to call my Mother-in-law "Ma." So, one day I said, "Ma, I think I'm ready to take the kids." She agreed. She said she wanted me to go visit her. We got a place in Windsor, and we did great! Life was great! It was awesome! We didn't have a TV for the first year, and we played games, and drew pictures, and we colored. All three of us agree that was the best year of our life. I went to school, and from grade eight into third year university. I was clean for five years. It was awesome! My Mom was so great. I have to give her so much credit. When I was in school, I could call her at 1 o'clock in the morning, and tell her I had a ten page essay that was due at eight o'clock in the morning. She would stay up all night with me, and she would help me do it over the phone. I didn't know the keyboard, and she would tell me where the letters were if I couldn't find them. Sometimes, the screen would go blank, and we'd have to start again. She helped me through all of them. I was trying to get my psych degree. She was really awesome!

But then, I relapsed again, when I bumped into an old friend. It was that, and I was working, and going to school full time, and single parenting my kids. I kind of really burned out! It was too much. Still I didn't have a diagnosis, or anything yet. I knew that something was wrong when I was in rehab. The cook in there would notice that I would forget how to do everything. She had a daughter who had A.D.D. She said to me once that she thought I had something called A.D.D. So I went to see a psychiatrist with them, and he diagnosed me as having severe A.D.H.D. So that gave me a diagnosis of something. So, that was the first time that I gave myself a break, and I wouldn't call myself down by telling myself I was an idiot, awful, you wreck families, or bad, or useless or anything. That was the first time that I said "Oh my God! There's something! I have a bit of a handicap in an area!" That gave me the courage to ask for help in university. I got a note taker, and I got extra time for my exams. That made my parents also realize that there was something wrong. They then noticed….and thought maybe she has something. It stopped being, "Why don't you stop doing this? Why did you do this? Will you keep doing this to us? Why do you keep doing this to yourself? Why do you keep doing this to other people? What are you thinking? What's the matter with you?" All the questions. It was a relief. The psychiatrist said that I was one of the worst cases he ever saw. I couldn't sit still for a minute. Every symptom all through school just matched the diagnosis of A.D.H.D.

After I relapsed, the kids had to go with Children's Services, and they stayed in a foster home for a year. Luckily, they went to an awesome one. They still talk to those foster parents. They took them on trips everywhere and treated them so well. I am grateful that it wasn't like any of the foster homes that I stayed in back in my day. I didn't have good experiences like they did. In that time of my kids being in foster care, I got pregnant with my son Eric. I was still living in Ontario. When I found out I was pregnant, I was thirty five years old, and I was almost four and a half months. It was a surprise, but it was a successful pregnancy. When he was a baby, he had to have open heart surgery. He is very intelligent, and a quiet person. He is the light of my life, and I love him to bits! I love all of my kids to bits!

I am doing great now. I work at Toys R Us now. I love it! I work on the baby side, and I am training new girls now. They understand. I was with an agency that helps you get jobs. It's a big agency, and they do job shadowing. I was going to interviews, but I wasn't getting any jobs. I snuck into an interview by myself at Toys R Us, and I got the job! I was slowly able to do good, and I was able to tell them that I don't have the best memory. They had no idea that it was FAS until we were on T.V. I hadn't told anyone, so it was a big surprise to everyone.

I moved to Calgary when my son was three years old. I was really lucky to get my diagnosis, because they were only taking five women that year. I met Dr. Liz Lawryk. It made me feel kind of sad once I got my diagnosis. It explained why my real Mom gave me up. It was a realization for everyone. However, within two weeks of my FAS diagnosis, Child Services took Eric away from me. They told me that I can't parent. They told me that I would have to live in supported living. It was a shock, because there weren't any problems. The diagnosis was good for me, because I gave myself a few more breaks. I didn't expect so much from myself anymore. I knew why I couldn't do things, and why I couldn't remember things. I stopped being so hard on myself. It took away the feeling that I was just a bad person. Things have been much easier since then. I have been able to get disability. I have been able to access so many programs. The bad thing was when they took my son, and they put him in Hull Homes. He was only five years old, and it wasn't easy for him. He was there for a year and a half. Child Services told me that I have to have a roommate that can help look after us. A lady named Sherry was able to help out, and we moved in with her. She was awesome! I was just at her house two days ago.

There was an agency called Closer to Home, and we had awful experiences with them. They said that we had to have their staff with us twenty four hours a day, and they were coming and going like our home was their office. They were supposed to be our support staff. There were forty two staff that we went through during our time with them. It was terrible! It was awful for Eric because they were strangers coming into our home, and it was constantly a different person. It was so invasive! We were the pilot project for that company. Eventually, we were able to get released from having to use their staff. I spoke to a lady, and told her my problems with everything, and through her, we were able arrange for someone to just drop in on us to check on how we were doing. They would come a couple times a week. Things have been good since then. My son is twelve years old now. He goes to tae kwon do. He's still very sweet, and he is doing alright.

I am doing different schedules with Toys R Us. I struggle with that a little bit now. I am going to Holland with my parents. I've been to Mexico many times. I have my grandson twice a week, because my daughter has gone back to work. I am a motivational speaker, and I go to schools to speak about it. My Mom does that with me too. I have a lot of things wrong with my body, like spinal stenosis. Liz wanted me to get a list of all of the things in my diagnosis, and to do a bunch of speaking. But I have problems with making phone calls, I didn't end up calling Liz back about all of the speaking engagements that she wanted me to do.

What is a normal life for you isn't normal for us. One thing to note, is that we may not be physically tired, but at the end of the day, we are mentally drained. Exhausted! Trying to live life, and deal with problems is hard. Mental strain is very much a problem for us. We are constantly trying to analyze what is being told to us or asked of us, so that we can understand. We have to overthink things. But one good thing is we never quit. No matter what situation we are in, we never quit.

ADVICE - *My advice for anyone who is struggling with FAS, my advice to them is to have support. I can't stress that enough. Be gentle to the ones who have FAS, because we have had had such a hard life. If you haven't been able to find support for you or your family, keep looking, because it is out there. There are more agencies out there, so don't give up. Life can be great, but you just can't give up!*

CHAPTER 6
Adrianna S.

I was born in 1994. My Mom was an alcoholic, but she was also doing cocaine, and she was a prostitute. My Mom and Dad were both drug addicts, to the point where I was in the hospital because my Mom had just had me, and he would try to sneak in cocaine. I was born a coke baby, because my Mom was an addict, authorities decided that they were going to put me straight into foster care.

I found out about all of this about my birth Mom when I was seventeen years old. I am in my twenties now. I knew I was different growing up, but she wanted me to wait until I was more mature. It hurts me to know that my Mom was a prostitute, and I was a cocaine baby, and they had to take me away. It was such a harsh struggle. I wasn't sure if I was an only child as well, but I found out that she had children before me. I have no idea where they are in their life. I got in contact with one of my biological brothers who is now sixteen. He told me that she now has a three year old. I could be a family of seven or eight. Everyone is going into foster care. It's hard to hear.

The hospital had put me into foster care, and my adoption became final when in 1997. My birth parents told me they lived constantly hoping that my new parents didn't want to take me. They had arrangements every weekend, but it all became final in 1997. That is when my new parents told them they didn't want that. They didn't want me to grow up confused. My real parents come for the weekend and be different from other structured parents. I don't remember anything about that, but growing up, my brother is special needs. He isn't my biological brother. My Mom adopted me because she couldn't have kids.

Growing up, being in elementary school, I remember failing classes. They never put me in summer school, because my parents didn't want to label me. They never treated me different or special assistance. I don't want to say I resent it, but in a way, I do. I thought I was really stupid. I hate the idea of that, and it breaks my heart now knowing what I know. I remember crying in class because I didn't understand. I remember in math class, she would call on me, and if I didn't know it, I would guess, and she would make fun of my guess. There are some cruel teachers out there. I would cry in class.

Sometimes, I over think, and I have really bad anxiety. I went to the doctors and told her about all of my worries. I shared about my FAS and being a cocaine baby. My doctor looked at me, and she told me that there is no way that I could be a cocaine baby, because it aborts the baby. She also told me I don't look like I have FAS. I told be talking about a carnival, and I would pop up and say something about a cat, for example. They would look at me as if to say you're weird! What's wrong with you? I had a lot of low self esteem issues. My parents were always very loving. My first seven years of my life were really terrible. There was a lot of abuse there. There was another sibling there that wasn't fine. The abuse I lived through really messed with me. I have had to carry that through my life. So, talking to people is hard. Talking to girls is hard. Being able to love is hard. I want to love, but because I can't always relate, I think I care about everyone more than I am able to love.

Academics were really hard. That is what led to me learning I have FAS. I didn't care much about education until probably ten years ago. It's like I woke up or something. I can research the heck out of anything now. Education was just hard for me. Learning was hard for me because I couldn't her to trust me and told her things about me like my eye sight, which is so bad. I can't focus, because my eyes focus differently. I have to pay so much more, because my lenses are so thick. But the doctor didn't listen to me, and it didn't help me even though I wanted help. Now, to help manage my anxiety, I go to the gym often. I feel like the gym gives me the best power to control my anxieties.

In elementary, school was hard, because I was aggressive, but I was also very loving and patient. I would lash out at my friends if something bothered me. I remember I was in the sand pit, I got upset, and I threw sand in my friend's face. I was very impatient. I would hit and slap, and it was because I couldn't voice what I was feeling. In high school, it was tough. With classes, they didn't have any special assistance, I failed almost every single class except for art. I went to summer school for about two years. I would beg my teachers to go into the learning room, to talk to one of the assistants. I had anxieties about school. I tried hard to keep up with other kids in school. I would cry before classes. The other kids were doing so well.

My parents sent me from a public school to a private academic Catholic school. I had no idea about the Catholic school system. They didn't have things like cooking class. They had things like science, math, religion. That kind of thing. The kids going into it were so intelligent. I remember at the end of every term, they would post everyone's grade average on the door, and I would be in the 50% range. My friends would complain about getting 93%. It was those things that gave me anxiety, that I didn't think I could do anything outside of school, I wasn't smart enough to get job. I had good friends. She was so smart. Sometimes it would bother me, because she would say things about getting a B, and it not being good enough. I loved high school in a way, but I felt like I didn't ever really fit in. I never had a relationship, and I didn't feel like I was mature. I still felt like a child. It took me a long time to do things. Now, I don't feel twenty one. I feel now would be around eighteen years old.

I got a job when I was nineteen in retail. I was working as a cashier, and it was the scariest thing I have done. I couldn't figure out the math, and people would be impatient, and ask if there was someone faster than me. It would make me so frustrated with myself, I would go to the back and cry, and end up quitting.

What I am doing now, I realize I really love children. I am enrolled to go to college in January. I am so excited. It will take three or four years for me to do Early Childhood Education. My job right now is a contact job. I would three days a week, from 7 to 5, and I get to be with kids. There is no anxiety with it, and the kids are so loving and always so happy to see me.

With relationships, sometimes I don't feel like I am mature enough to have a relationship. Sometimes, I expect people to feel the same way I feel, or to think how I think. My parents divorced when I was sixteen, and I hated it. I felt my parents didn't have a stable household. My Dad is an impatient person, and he would get mad at me, and ask me, "Why don't you get this?" or "Why don't you understand this?" He would compare me to other kids my age. I think with anyone who has FAS, I hope that they have a stable home. My Mom and her boyfriend go to California for six months at a time. I am trying to see if I can get a social worker. Someone who can just stay in contact with me. I went on YouTube a few months ago. I was so desperate to find support and learn more about FAS. I found a guy named Morgan Fawcette. He is a First Nations man who lives with FASD. I got in touch with him, and he said he would look into some supports. I am still waiting on that too. I have always thought maybe I could become a speaker, since finding out about my FAS and cocaine addiction as a baby. I would definitely want to support anyone who has gone through any of this. It is nice to be able to agree that I went through high school and I couldn't understand things like other normal kids. It was super frustrating, and the depression that comes with that. I wish that I had a counselor, because I felt feelings that I could never talk to my parents about. I have not had a formal diagnosis, but I did look into it. The price I was quoted is not a price that I can afford. I have been noted as having FAS since I was a baby, but not a formal diagnosis.

I am going through the beginning journey to learn more about myself. I have wanted to get in contact with my birth parents. I want to know how I look most like. I want to know if there are pictures of me when I was a baby. I want to know if my parents knew what they were letting happen to me when she was pregnant with me. There are things that I want to know to fill in gaps.

ADVICE - My advice for other people who are learning about FAS. I have never had any issues with alcohol or drugs. I have been good with staying away from it. I stay away from parties, but I have had a few bad experiences. I don't want that in my life. Stay away from the things that can bring you into a downward spiral. Take moments for yourself. Going to the gym or take up a hobby so you have your own focus away from anxiety is a big help. Having a good support system is also very good. At the end of a hard day, my boyfriend gives me a hug, and it takes away the edge off my anxiety too.

CHAPTER 7
Christopher H.

In the 70's, it was called FAS. I wanted to share the positive of living with FAS. We hear about all of the negative aspects living with FAS. It is so overwhelming having to live with it.

I didn't know about my FAS until a little over a year ago. It was a week before my 44th birthday last May. My Dad told me last year about having FAS. It was through a causal conversation, and we were just talking. It was really just a misunderstanding, but it was also something that I kind of already knew. My brother blew a full 4-year scholarship to university, but he is a genius. I always hated the fact that he never had to open a book or work so hard to learn anything. I told my Dad that, and he said, "Well, you know why that is?" I told him I didn't. He said to me, "You were born with fetal alcohol syndrome." He told me that he had to search high and low because they wanted to know what was going on, because we needed to help you. My Dad is a retired doctor now, he had more avenues, and so he was able to share this with me. He thought that my Mom told me, and she had never.

I was adopted. I was the only one who was adopted out. I was taken from my mother. She had tuberculosis, and I had tuberculosis. Then I was in a foster family for seven years. Then I was adopted. I was adopted at the age of seven. When I was around twelve years of age, I found a birth certificate while I was looking for something in my parent' room. I came across this birth certificate. It had my name, and my birth parents. It also had written a note, "some known use of alcohol". I took it, and I carried it with me for years. I realized, at the time, I was thinking it was a fancy way of saying that she was just an alcoholic.

However, what I have noticed in my life is what my parents taught me has served me well up until this point. My life has been hell, but I have been able to overcome so many things. I have been through a lot of stuff, and it is truly amazing that I am blessed today. I don't think I am any different than any other people. I have just learned different ways to cope with what I have. I live better now than I ever have in my whole life. I had to make some changes. I have had girlfriends that have helped me make those changes. My parents never left me. I lost touch with my parents a little bit over the years, but we recently became re-acquainted. My parents live in California, and I live in Missouri. Before I moved here, I was moving a lot. From one state – a frying pan, to another state – another frying pan. Between those two moves, I lost everything. I got burned! I had been struggling for a few months. I was made to help others, but I don't have a means to be able to do so. So, it has been a bit frustrating. Being able to tell my story is my way to help others who have FAS.

After I found out, I must have watched every single video on YouTube, and read, and looked up as much as I could on the internet. Even some groups up in Canada. It was overwhelming. I was learning about myself in a way that was very real. The struggles that I was going throughout my life are many.

Elementary school years, as a kid, I was socially awkward. I didn't know how the world works around me. When people are talking or sharing stories, I have a hard time responding, because I don't get it. I don't relate. So, to cope, I have memorized how to relate, but I really don't feel the same. I have always been there. It's kind of disturbing, because I want to be there with you on your level. It can up and down. I just seem to have a hard time connecting. I would say awkward things, out of context. Someone would

do it. Oh man! My Dad and I would go rounds!!! Not rounds, but you know what I mean! When doing school work, I would get responses from my Dad like, "You know better than that! You're smarter than that! We've been through this!" Math was hard! When I read that math can be a real issue for some people who have FAS, I was like wow!! When I found out, I was happy about it! Just for that moment! I may use my fingers to subtract, but I love algebra! I love calculus, and all those things! I like physics. I did try college, but it was really very imbalanced for me. I was always struggling to balance. It sometimes caused a lot of problems for me.

I have had my share of institutions. I've been to jail. I have had my share of that! I have also had my share of suicide attempts. Like I said, I am very blessed to be alive. I used to think of suicide all the time. I don't now why. I have hurt a lot of people. Not intentionally. Emotionally, the desire to not want to live can be so overwhelming. I just couldn't seem to figure out how to live life. I really wanted to learn how to live. I moved here to Missouri in April 2013. I stayed with some friends. It took time for me to get settled. I went through some really hard times, but now, I wake up every day, and think about what is going to be my motivation for that day. I have to take time to think about what I am going to do. I recently made the change to not beat myself up for what I am not. I thought for a long time that I should have been something because everyone else was. I now accept what I am today. I do things that make me happy. I do a lot of art. I do fiber arts. It keeps me busy. I tinker with electronics. I don't like being cluttered. My whole life seemed to be so chaotic. I don't like clutter. I don't press myself about who I think I need to be. I think God will let me know when it is to happen. I have a good church family now. I take one step at a time.

During my youth, and adult years, I did struggle with addictions. I don't know. I was terribly abused for a lot of years, and I know that my use of all of that…that is what that was about. I was concealing the pain of the early years. I began drinking when I was fifteen. It controlled me for many years. I met my mother. She's an alcoholic. I have met some siblings too. I have four half-brothers, and one adopted brother. They all have their issues. I went through a stage when I wondered about what my purpose was. What am I supposed to be doing with my life? It really got me! However, I went through some things in my life that have brought me to where I am right now. I went through my life and the challenges always thinking that I was always doing something wrong or going to do something wrong. It becomes so tiring. It was the constant message that I was always receiving though, so I became conditioned to believe that I was bad. I went through the program, and fell off, and stayed sober, and then fell off again. I am a human being first, but I don't think I have ever really blamed anyone. I think I blame God more than anyone. My natural mother wasn't raised well. She wasn't educated. She had the very bare minimum. I am the second person in that entire family who has graduated and gone to college in my natural family. My brothers all dropped out. I have one brother who has died. I'm not sure how he died.

Throughout my life, I have lived with fear, anxiety, lack of confidence, and not liking myself. I never knew where to go. I have been afraid of everything. When I found God, all of that was gone. Through everything I have come through, I now look at how I am able to help other people more clearly now. My advice? You're blessed. Look at the positive and keep putting one foot in front of the other. Support is really important. Finding good people who you can go to when things get a bit rough is important. I am blessed, and I am grateful to have gone through all of my struggles. I have been diagnosed with disorders, and we are now looking into the possibility of autism. Finding out about FAS has provided a lot of answers. It is a blessing in disguise.

ADVICE – *Relying on my faith and my family has helped me. I know I am blessed even though I have gone through so many struggles. Answers will come. You just have to start searching them out.*

CHAPTER 8
Rodney James – (RJ) F.

I love the reasons why you are writing this book! It is the exact same reasons that I do what I do. When I got my diagnosis, I had to teach myself about FASD! It was kind of like, "Yup! You've got it! Thanks for coming out!" And I'm like, well….what is it? When I asked that, they gave me nothing! Seriously! Nothing! No supports! No information! I had a pamphlet, and that was it! It was really, really depressing. When I went online, I was reading stuff, and Bonnie Buxton's book saved my life. Her book is called Damaged Angels. When I read that book, there was hope. Umm, I haven't had the chance to meet her daughter or Bonnie yet, but I have seen them both speaking, and they were exactly what I needed. From that point, it was kind of like I had to say something! I can't keep quiet anymore! So, I started my Facebook group, which is my first tentative little step into talking to the public. I believe we are the largest FASD support and FASD information group on Facebook. We have some really incredible people there. They are part of the group, and they really do pay attention. In 2011 – 2012, it was a little sketchy. On February 14th, that is the day I went public with it. When I launched the group on February 14th, I figured maybe twenty people might join. It would just be a few of us going wow! Life has been unfair. We are the people who are ignored, because most times, out disability is invisible. When you're invisible, it's kind of like well! What are we going to do? When I started this group, people started listening! So, I just started continuing with it. I knew it was being picked up on blogs, and suddenly I was attracting other like-minded people. More people were joining. Jody Kulp, who is from Minnesota, has been instrumental in a lot of things that happened.

I then ended up going to the AG-7 conference. I went there three years ago now, as a guest. Somebody sponsored me to go there, and there I began to make more contacts. I did a little speaking there. It picked up from there. The next thing I know, I was sponsored to take the FASD certificate course. Since I got out of school when I finished in August, it's been almost non-stop. I took 3 months off last winter. I even had a heart attack this September, which slowed me down! I had to take 6 weeks off, but as soon as the six weeks were over, I was back on the road and the AG -7 was my first show back. It was supposed to be my last show of the season, but I have 1 more this weekend in my hometown! I have never spoken there. It's going to be interesting, because these are my relatives!

A little bit about my background. I was born in Ontario on October 13th, 1961 to an unwed mother. She was First Nations. My mom had been part of the residential school system for a couple of for a few years, until my grandmother found out what was going on. When your reserve is right beside a town, and you have Native school, local kids can, if they can't make it to the residential school, can make it into town. It was a very rare thing, so my mother was pulled out. She had been attending residential school for three years, and she was left handed. They told her it was the hand of the devil, and they tied her left hand behind her back, so she was forced to use her right hand. They did dental procedures with no anesthetic for the pain. So, my mother had her issues because of her experiences in the residential school. Of course, my grandfather had been through residential school system. His entire teen years, so he had his own issues. My grandmother hadn't! My grandmother didn't drink, but while a lot of the effects on my family looked like it could be FASD, I think that they are trauma based. I was born into an extremely traumatized family. Society at that time, disappearing Indian was a real possibility. In fact, my grandmother even stopped teaching anything about being Native. I was about eight years old, and she told me that we were a disappearing people, and so to teach me anything, there was no point. They were defeated and fighting amongst themselves to survive. That is what I lived with. That type of environment and society. The racial tensions between the town and where I grew up may have been greater for other people, but I was able to make the transition almost seamlessly. That wasn't a big deal. There was a lot of sadness on the reserve.

So, my mother had me, and she actually gave me up at birth! My grandmother took me at birth. They didn't actually adopt me, but they fostered me. They kept me for over three years, at which point my mother re-married, and the gentleman she married said he would adopt me, and that's why I have this fine Polish last name! I do have two sisters from that marriage, and they were together for about four or five years. They both drank. With the drinking, they used to fight. It was kind of horrifying! I still call him my father, and I made the conscious choice to keep this last name. My mother eventually left my father, took us, and we moved around a lot. That's quite common with that type of situation. She remarried a few times. I remember Uncles and things like that. Through to this point, there has been all kind of physical and emotional abuse, as well as sexual abuse going on. It wasn't happening all the time, but it happened enough to not be something that was extraordinary or unusual kind of thing. So, we went back to my grandmothers. My mother had disappeared, and she had been gone for over a week. I phone grandmother up, and I said we need some food. So, she came and got us, and she took us in. I wasn't the same! My grandparents went through hell from the family. They didn't understand! The reserve didn't understand! They thought I was some little kid who was parachuted in from nowhere. When you're an illegitimate child born in the 1960's, Mom hides!! Very few people even knew that I had been born! I couldn't even take the reserve bus! I wasn't allowed. I had to take another bus from another reserve that passed through our reserve. That was the only bus I could take! I used to get bullied on that bus too. They'd tie up my arms, and tie me to the seat, and then I would have to take the bus all the way around the route! They didn't hurt me. They just did these really annoying things! It wasn't a horrible experience though.

As a child with FASD, I was sexually precocious. It had already been experienced through whatever I had been through. By the age of twelve, I had figured out how to get much older women! I will leave it at that. By the age of

137

fourteen, I was already in trouble with the law. It was me doing car breaks in, and home break ins. I don't know why, but I also had a thing with climbing. I loved climbing! I had this thing with climbing buildings! I loved going up to the second or the third floor! I would jump from roofs! I don't know if I thought I was comic book character, but I was just in my wild, and crazy teenage years. Going back – physical issues that I had growing up, and one which I like to tell people is that one of my legs is shorter than the other! I had balance issues, scoliosis, floppy joints, I've dislocated many joints. Early on, I had an opportunity to go into martial arts. In martial arts, you have to build core body strength, that's how I hold myself together. Exercise is very important to me! I take melatonin to help me sleep. I take vitamins due to the issues that I experience now. During the formation in the mother, the alcohol depletes the nutrition which would otherwise be absorbed.

So, I ended up in a position where I was going to a group home. The reason I went to a group home was during that period between my grandmother and the group home, approximately twelve months, I went through about thirteen foster homes. I'd like to say it was the foster parents fault, but that would be a lie! I was not easy to get along with. I was the proverbial "wild child." As a child, the behavior I was exhibiting was passive aggression. You could say whatever you wanted to me and I would say yes or no, but I would still do whatever I wanted. It wasn't malicious. If I was ever confronted, I would be very reactive. If you come at me in a positive, wholesome way, I will mirror that. But if you come at me ready to fight, or are confrontational, I'll mirror that. It was fight or flight! I'm used to having to defend myself. Being reactive got me in a lot of trouble. For the most part, even though I was the one who was being told that I was all sorts of things by psychologists, and doctors and having had all assessments done and who were all telling me I was this, this and this. I have this whole list of problems which I call alphabet soup diagnosis, I kept feeling that they were wrong. Of course, that's classic! If you're crazy, you don't know you're crazy. I was hearing that I had A.D.H.D, OCD, ODD, PTSD, reactive attachment disorder, and they assessed me to see if I was psychotic. They even went as far as to test me for being a sociopath. It's insulting to think that people may think that you're a sociopath, or even worse! A psychopath! They spend a lot of money testing me. These were a couple of the words I heard. I understand that! But on another level, I've always spoken to animals, and they talk to me. I can understand that. That's a thought process that works. I know I'm not defective, because I can understand animals. It's human beings I have a problem with! I took computer programming in grade ten. We're talking punch cards, and programming from a thousand years ago! The programming they taught me made sense. A goes to B goes to C. If not, then it goes to here and here. You could see it charted out like that. That kind of thing made sense to me, and that is my thought process. Human beings are totally different! I couldn't understand them! But they were telling me all of this, and I was reacting in a very passive aggressive way. I would respond to them by telling them that I wasn't like they were saying I was. Nobody would listen even though I would bring it up. This was my first year of speaking. So, feeling that the diagnosis that I was hearing, it fit into fueling my passive aggressive behavior. I am bullheaded. It must be the Scottish in me. I know they're wrong! But there was no point in fighting it, so I buried it more or less. It was just something that I dealt with.

After grade nine, I quit school. During the summer of grade nine, I had been involved in a car accident, so when I went back to start grade ten, I was on crutches. Grade ten didn't work out. I last about four months. I was also caught standing outside smoking! In school, there were some things that I loved. I ended up doing double English and double History in grade nine in place of math and science. I have no idea how I worked that out! I managed to do the same thing in Sea Cadets too. There I was Sea Clerk, and we had run out of Petty officers. I found a little loop hole that said someone could substitute someone as an acting petty officer. By the time I had left, I was an acting Chief Petty Officer, but I was actually only a leading cadet. That's three or four ranks below! I was the one doing the paper work! I always knew I wasn't as stupid as people tended to tell me I was.

I grew up. Life has a tendency to make that happen! When my son was born, I had the same vicious dysfunctional cycle going on in my life that I knew had to end. The same horrible one that I saw growing up. Part of that ending was me changing who I was, what I did and everything surrounding that. I needed to change the intergenerational cycle of abuse. I needed to become a responsible adult, although I never quite succeeded in that part of it, but I sometimes played one on TV!! That was a formative change in my life because I took responsibility at that point with me going to college. I never graduated, but I went, and I took broadcasting. Because of only one thing, and this is what I tell people! I had a talent for photography. Some people like my voice, and it was continuously suggested as a career option. I'd hear, "You should go into radio!" Well, I thought I was, and I did the TV thing, which is part of it. I did it more or less for fun! I picked up a camera, because I liked to shoot! I would do projects. I won three awards for my photography, so instead of going into radio, I went into television as a photographer. I followed my own talents. I did that for almost twenty years. I did eighteen years as a shooter, and a year and half directing news casts at CTV. I had an entire career doing that.

I got married. My daughter was born. I got divorced, and my entire life fell apart. The relationship of my marriage was about ten years. We were married for just about five years. I went to work one day, I came back, and there was no furniture in the house. It was very abrupt. She didn't explain why. However, when we were together, she would fulfill the role of being my external brain. I fell apart completely! I went through anger management. I would try anything! Yes, of course I'm angry, but under that, I was very, very hurt. I gave my photography up when I went through my divorce. I rarely ever pick up a camera now. I did do a video at the conference, with the odd shot here and there. I sailed through the anger management course because that wasn't the problem. The problem was that it ended up being more about what she wanted than anything else. I tried! It got to the point where I had to leave Sudbury, which is where I was living at the time. I came back to Thunderbay. I could have tried to get a job back here at the station, but instead I lost my mind, and became a truck driver! I took the course, and I became a long-haul truck driver. I had about 750,000 kms of road under my belt, but I had a disagreement with the landing gear on my truck. I was reefing and pulling on the landing gear, and there were two ligaments that were torn off my spinal cord. The tear actually took two pieces of bone with them! So, I get to say my back's broken in two places!! It's not major, but it did keep me on my back for about two years. That happened in 2003 or 2004. During that period, a woman who I had been dating had decided that we weren't working out. We are still friends. She kept saying to me that she kept reading about this thing called FAS. She said to me, "I think it might fit!" Now, I was going into some severe depression anyways, and I had tried to kill myself. I was admitted to the hospital. I was confined to a hospital by a doctor. I was locked up for eight days, and that was enough. Especially when a big part of the ward population is suffering from other mental illnesses. During that time, that's when I was referred to a psychiatrist. That is when he began to finally agree with me about the diagnosis in the past not all fitting. We went through all of them. He listened to my concerns. We reviewed all of them, and I was able to point out the major discrepancies. I brought up the idea of FAS with him, and he was very up front with me, and told me, "I have no idea what that is!" That was in 2007. So that is what he had to work with. The big blue diagnostics manual that they use didn't even have FAS in there. I brought him Bonnie Buxton's book in. He read it, and he said, "You know? I really don't understand!" He then referred me for a diagnosis. The diagnosis for adults wasn't done in Thunderbay. So, I'm the first adult to be diagnosed in Thunderbay. We now do them quite regularly. I set up a support group through Norwest Health Centre, which is where I got my diagnosis. So, we have a support group there now, and I run the adult support group now. The people who get a diagnosis are given an option to come, and we try to inform them. That is sort of how I ended up on the track to where I am now. Proving the maternal drinking was rather difficult because my Mother died. She drank until she died of pancreatic cancer. It was more than likely caused by the drinking. She had already passed, but I was able to get an aunt that had been around at that time who was able to speak to the past, and she was able to confirm it the maternal drinking. Through St. Michael's hospital in Thunderbay through a teleconference, the diagnosis was confirmed. It took about five years altogether. Through the research, they dug up the most incredible school records. I have my kindergarten report card! In the first term, I failed math! I failed math time!! Apparently, I would lay down, and I wouldn't stay on task, and I was a holy terror! The research found the most incredible stuff! Once I got my diagnosis, it was kind of like, "Ok! What do we do now?" I went home, but it just didn't sit right with me. I did some research, and everything was so cut in stone, and so depressing!! It was quite bleak! The information I had didn't outline if people who had FAS had a future! That made me angry! Part of the ancillary testing as part of the diagnosis, I was able to complete some genetic testing done. The technician who presented the findings decided to throw in on his own that he wouldn't shoot a pregnant woman for having a glass or wine or two, if she wanted to. That was in 2010. It's a human failing. If we enjoy it, we make excuses and allowances. Drinking is something that is normalized, and that is enjoyed. I have met people who are on the complete opposite side of the spectrum with a zero tolerance for alcohol. We can't do that either. We have to find that acceptable tolerance of use.

The next year I spoke, I said if you know one person with FASD, then you know one person with FASD. We are so brilliantly different! I find it hard to speak for everyone or as a group. There are somethings that we share similarities, but we are the most incredibly diverse and vibrant group of people I know! I love working with adults who have FASD. There's challenges, but we get through those. I guess I am a late bloomer! I'm doing what I love! I thought I was successful doing television! I was working in Prague for and ABC affiliate network. One day, I was looking around, and I remember thinking, "Where do I go from here?" So, I thought that I had done everything in my life. I have been given an incredible new lease on life! That heart attack, although it slowed me down, we have almost 100% confirmation that it was a birth defect. It is related to the FASD. Now we know that the FASD damage tends to be in the spinal cord and it goes almost straight down. A heart problem had been detected when I was about sixteen and trying to get into the military. This intermittent heart problem only showed up twice in between. Every time I go for an EKG, I come back with a clean heart check. There were these two incidents in my adult life which showed up. On September 4th of this year, I woke up and it decided to show itself one more time. I had a stint put in that day. The damage was quite minimal. I'm on meds for a year now. Within three days, they allowed me to go back to my regular exercise routine. It totally confused them at Cardio Care when I showed them how much I do. So, cardio was over for me. I didn't get to walk on the treadmill or anything this time. It's actually been the best heart attack anyone could have. I'm still weak, but I'm working on that. I get better all the time. It was horrible though, because I had two presentations on September 9th. I will try again next year.

My very first speaking engagement came about shortly after my diagnosis. I asked while I was at the Norwest Regional Center. They have an FASD event every year. That particular year, a prominent occupational therapist named Kim Bartel was speaking. I asked if I could take part in this event. They accepted my request to be part of the event, and they let me introduce her. I did a small five minute speech, which I still have on YouTube. I think it was one of my most embarrassing speeches ever! My first public speech was in front of about 250 people. I dressed up nice, and I took my paper. They had vetted my speech, word for word. They told me to not deviate, and that I only had this amount of time.

So, I read my speech. I hate it every time I see that first speech, I cringe! My head was down, and it wasn't what I wanted. The message was me, but the energy wasn't. But overall, I liked people listening to me! I think it's the old man in me! At a certain point, you just decide that people should listen to you. Now, I am able to gather them into a room, close the doors so they're stuck there, and they have to listen to me!!! For an old man, that's a perfect dream!

I know that there's a segment of our population that are neuro-typical and non-neurotypical, who just accept someone talking to you rather than just reading something. Part of it is about meeting people and going to see people face to face. I worked in television long enough to pick up a few tricks about things that you should have to do. I have made my initials "R.J." into a brand almost. From there, I just started selling it! People started listening and it is had grown. I sometimes get invited to speak at events now, rather than go out and send abstract queries to go to events. My red shoes are part of my personality quirk. I was looking around, and there was nothing that set me apart from anyone, and it became problematic for me. I wanted to stand out. I chose the red shoes, and I hadn't seen high tops for a long time. I saw the pair of Converse, and I had to have them. I liked how they looked with my suit! Red is the color of the heart, the color of blood. It's vibrant and bright, and everybody has to wear shoes. It was a simple way to bring everybody together! So, now it has become if you're wearing red shoes, you're supporting us!

I was honored by being able to be the first speaker, and this year they let all four of me and my friends open. There are four of us that sit on panel, and we have become like family. The conference that I went to is getting larger and larger. I believe the last one had almost 400 people in attendance. Support and education is where the growth is, and this is where we need people. This is where we need the money, even if it means educating other adults. The pragmatic reality for adults my age who have FASD, is that there are no statistics or much information. It's sad to know, but quite often, people who have FASD don't live a long life.

At my last conference, people were talking about my personality. I'm kind of out there, and I am an extrovert. I have always been able to do that. In the past, however, it was a false bravado. It was like a mask I was wearing to disguise how I really felt, and so I would try to impress people, and was always trying to be the life of the party. I have the gift of gab, and I was always the class clown. It was always there. But as I was telling them at the conference now, I have self-confidence. I have more self-confidence now! I am even amazing myself sometimes, when I know thing that I don't know how I know. When people ask me stuff and this stuff comes out of me so naturally, the little me inside me that is running the machine back there is like, "What???" Where is the information coming from?? It's amazing what I know now! Having the freedom and the confidence to allow that to happen is a good feeling. All of my life I have had people tell me I was bad, I was crazy. I couldn't tell people what was happening inside my brain. I didn't want to tell people what was going on inside my brain! I was seeing things, and figuring things out, but I was afraid to say anything. But I'm not anymore. That's why I am a motivational speaker.

ADVICE - *Advice for people who are learning about FASD or who need encouragement. An elder told me that as a First Nations people, we understand that because we are born with this condition, we leave a part of us in the spirit world, and we maintain the connection to the Creator. That is our purpose. Society might try to make us feel less connected, but we are fully connected human beings. We are part of the human race. We are the ones who make it all happen. And remember, if you know one person with FASD, then you know one person with FASD!! And if you wear red shoes, then you are supporting us!*

FASD Online Resources

There are numerous resources available within the cities across Canada. I have listed a few of the provincial government web pages which contain more specific information to help you begin your own research.

Government of Canada -

https://www.canada.ca/en/public-health/services/diseases/fetal-alcohol-spectrum-disorder/support.html

British Columbia -

https://www2.gov.bc.ca/gov/content/health/managing-your-health/healthy-women-children/child-behaviour-development/special-needs/fetal-alcohol-spectrum-disorder-fasd

Alberta - http://fasd.alberta.ca/

Saskatchewan -
https://www.saskatchewan.ca/residents/health/a
ccessing-health-care-services/health-services-
for-people-with-disabilities/fetal-alcohol-
spectrum-disorder-services

Manitoba -
https://www.gov.mb.ca/healthychild/fasd/

Ontario -
http://www.children.gov.on.ca/htdocs/English/s
pecialneeds/fasd/index.aspx

Quebec -
http://www.ementalhealth.ca/Quebec/Fetal-
Alcohol-Spectrum-Disorders-
FASD/index.php?m=article&ID=14858

Newfoundland -

http://www.ementalhealth.ca/Newfoundland-
and-Labrador/Fetal-Alcohol-and-Fetal-Alcohol-
Spectrum-Disorders-
FASD/index.php?m=heading&ID=39

Prince Edward Island -

http://primarycare.ementalhealth.ca/Prince-
Edward-Island/Fetal-Alcohol-Spectrum-
Disorders-
FASD/index.php?m=article&ID=14858

Nova Scotia -

https://www.vitalitenb.ca/en/points-
service/mental-health/new-brunswick-fetal-
alcohol-spectrum-disorder-fasd-centre-
excellence/nb-fasd-centre-excellence

Yukon -

http://www.hss.gov.yk.ca/FASDplan.php

Northwest Territories -

http://services.exec.gov.nt.ca/service/433

Nunavut -

https://www.pauktuutit.ca/health/fetal-alcohol-spectrum-disorder/

ABOUT THE
AUTHOR

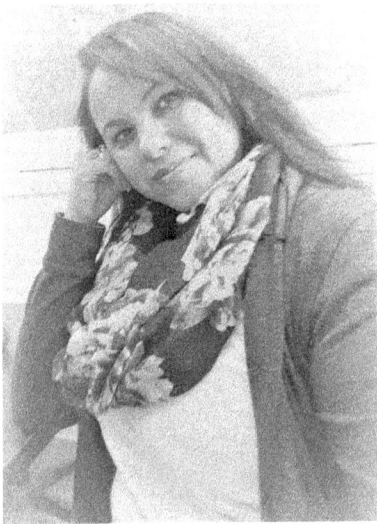

Charlene Trudel, a Kaska Dena from the Liard First Nation, was adopted as a young girl and is the youngest of four children. She grew up in rural northern British Columbia on a hobby farm, which instilled a love of nature and the outdoors. After completing high school, she moved to Kamloops in 1996 to study psychology. In 2000, she moved to Alberta where she met her handsome husband. Since moving to Alberta, she has made her career within the oil and gas industry and is currently completing a degree in Justice Studies. She resides in Calgary with her family, two spoiled cats, a pudgy guard dog, and has two grandchildren.

For further information, you can contact the author at charlenep93@gmail.com.

ABOUT THE PUBLISHER

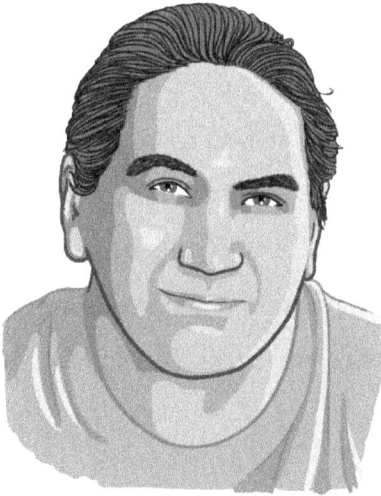

Only a few short years after the *Occupation of Alcatraz,* the *Wounded Knee Incident* and the *Shootout at Pine Ridge Reservation,* a boy was conceived.

Born in Seattle, raised on four reservations and in two cities, Jason EagleSpeaker is both Blackfoot and Duwamish. He is an award winning internationally esteemed author, graphic novelist and indie publisher. His hard hitting true stories focus on revealing Indigenous peoples' modern experiences.

Looking to publish your book, collaborate on a children's book or find more of Jason's books? You can easily connect with him online through social media, or email: jason@eaglespeaker.com or via his website - **www.eaglespeaker.com** (join his awesome email list while you're there).

MORE FROM EAGLESPEAKER PUBLISHING

NAPI CHILDREN'S BOOKS:

Napi and the Rock

Napi and the Bullberries

Napi and the Wolves

Napi and the Buffalo

Napi and the Chickadees

Napi and the Coyote

Napi and the Elk

Napi and the Gophers

Napi and the Mice

Napi and the Bobcat

Napi and The Jump

Napi: The Anthology

… and many more

GRAPHIC NOVELS:

UNeducation: A Residential School Graphic Novel

Napi the Trixster: A Blackfoot Graphic Novel

UNeducation, Vol 2

COLLABORATIONS:

The Great Cheyenne

The Empowerment of Eahwahewi

Descendants of Warriors

Hello … Fruit Basket

How The Earth Was Created

I Am The Opioid Crisis

My Ribbon Skirts

Real Indian

The Secret of the Stars

Scared – Coming Full Circle

Aahksoyo'p Nootski Cookbook

… and many many more

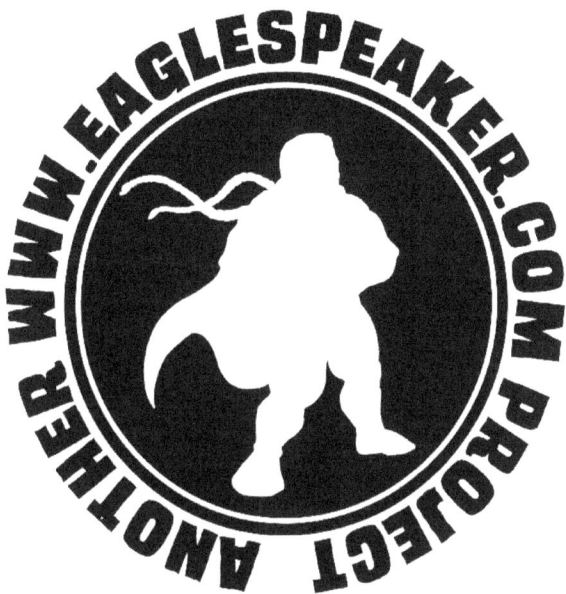

** If you absolutely loved this book, please tell your friends, then find it on AMAZON.COM and leave a quick review. Your words help more than you may realize. Thanks so much.

For bulk orders, and more Indigenous awesomeness, visit **www.eaglespeaker.com**

CPSIA information can be obtained
at www.ICGtesting.com
Printed in the USA
LVHW031453251118
598200LV00009B/225/P

9 781720 790600